Exploring Interrelationships between Fine Art and Nursing

Hazel Mary Cope MAVA Hons. (First Class), R.N. Certified Midwife,

Diploma in Tropical Disease Nursing, Cert. Cardio Thoracic Nursing

Queensland College of Art, Arts, Education and Law

Griffith University

Submitted in partial fulfilment of the requirements of the

Degree of

Doctor of Visual Art

March 2016

STATEMENT OF ORIGINALITY:

This work has not previously been submitted for a degree or diploma in any university. To the best of my knowledge and belief, the thesis contains no material previously published or written by another person except where due reference is made in the thesis itself.

Hazel Mary Cope   **March 2016**
___________________________   _______________
Hazel Mary Cope   Date

Abstract

The nursing profession can be characterised as a unique blend of attributes and philosophies that encompass scientific knowledge and artistic process. The interpersonal experience of caring in nursing is associated with a positivist sense of expression, acute observation, and compassion. It shares with artistic experience an intense motivation and analysis that involve the creative engagement of the senses. This research is informed by my forty-six years of working as a practicing registered nurse, and it takes an interdisciplinary approach between fine arts and nursing science to explore the elusive qualities of the human caring experience. My studio exploration, which uses everyday objects from the medical arena, highlights the values of empathy and sensitivity that are fundamental to the nurse–patient relationship. This is achieved through the formal strategies of repetition and placing everyday medical items in unfamiliar contexts, subsequently transforming them to evoke a provocative visual experience. These everyday items become a conduit for viewers to experience a new sensation. Functional objects are elevated to the poetic, enabling meanings to emerge that circumvent utilitarian and common associations. This research also highlights the impact of advancing technology and increased time pressures on the contemporary context of nursing, and the effect this has in decreasing interpersonal relations between nurse and patient. Furthermore, this project seeks to support interdisciplinary collaboration between visual arts and nursing science as a means to gain a better understanding of both disciplines. In doing so, I make no grandiose claims for either art or nursing as sole purveyors of feeling and emotion, but rather seek to examine the connections and correspondences between these two areas of practice that both seem to function from an underlying assumption that human beings have an unspoken desire to engage with each other.

TABLE OF CONTENTS

Page

List of Figures   5

Acknowledgements   7

Introduction   8

Chapter 1: Nursing and the Visual Arts   12

Chapter 2: Exploring the Research Question   17

Chapter 3: Time and Technology   21

Chapter 4: The Everyday in Nursing and Art   25

Chapter 5: Contextual Review   31

Chapter 6: Studio Practice   43

Chapter 7: Conclusion   74

Appendix   76

References   79

Bibliography   83

List of Figures

Unless otherwise noted, all works are by Hazel Mary Cope.

Figure		**Page**
1.	Hendrick Terbruggen *St. Sebastian Attended by St. Irene* 1625, oil on canvas, 149 x 119.4cm. Collection of Allen Memorial Art Museum, Oberlin, Ohio.	12
2.	Anonymous *The Old Style Nurse* 1879, cartoon. The Mansell Collection, London.	12
3.	Thomas Eakins *The Agnew Clinic* (detail) 1889, oil on canvas, 213 x 335cm. Collection of Philadelphia Museum of Art.	14
4.	Novelty nurse costume 2013	15
5.	Book cover, 1950s	15
6.	*This Will Hurt!* 2009 pastel on paper, 55 x 35cm	19
7.	*Voided 500mls* 2009, pastel on paper 55 x 35cm	19
8.	Germaine Koh *Knitwork* 1992–ongoing	21
9.	Robert Pope *Chemotherapy* 1989, acrylic on canvas, 61 x 91.4cm. Robert Pope Foundation.	31
10	Robert Pope *Sparrow* 1989, acrylic on canvas, 61 x 76.2cm. Robert Pope Foundation.	32
11	Robert Pope *Mountain* 1990, acrylic on canvas, 91.4 x 132.2cm. Robert Pope Foundation.	33
12	Rebecca Horn *Finger Gloves* 1972, fabric, wood, and metal. Tate Collection.	35
13.	Richard Prince *Nurse of Greenmeadow* 2002, inkjet print and acrylic on canvas, 228.6 x 266.7cm. Private collection.	37
14.	William Kentridge *Drawing from Stereoscope,* 1998–99, charcoal, pastel, and coloured pencil, 120 x 160cm. Collection of Museum of Modern Art, New York.	39
15.	Michael Elmgreen and Ingar Dragset *Please, Keep Quiet!* 2003, installation. Collection of Statens Museum for Kunst, National Gallery of Denmark.	41
16.	*Enough Is Enough* 2009, pastel on paper, 55 x 35cm	43
17.	*Hand Study* 2009, potassium permanganate on canvas, 92 x 122cm	44
18.	*Soft Conduit* 2009, potassium permanganate on canvas, 122 x 92cm	44
19.	*Florence Pringle* 2011, watercolour and potassium permanganate on canvas, 92 x 122cm	44
20.	*X-ray* 2011, charcoal on paper, 50 x 40cm	45
21.	*I Should Really Wear Gloves But I Can't Feel Your Veins* 2009, pastel on paper, 50 x 40cm	46
22.	*Our Nurses* 2009, mixed media with needles and gauze, 10 x 8cm	47
23.	Gold Coast City Art Gallery 2009	48
24.	*Nurse's Coif* 2008, digital photograph	49
25.	*Nurse's Coif and Surgical Instruments* 2009, digital photograph	50
26.	*Fan1* 2010, digital photograph	51
27.	*Butterfly* 2010, digital photograph	52
28.	*No. 42 Waiting* 2010, digital photograph	53
29.	*Untitled* 2011, digital photograph	53
30.	*Blade Holder* 2013, surgical instruments mounted on wood, 70 x 85cm	54

31. *Heart Starter* 2013, surgical instruments mounted on wood, 70 x 85cm   54
32. *Mandala* 2013, surgical instruments mounted on wood, 85 x 85cm   55
33. *Absence and Presence* 2014, gauze squares sewn together with silk, 1500 x 2400cm   58
34. *Absence and Presence* 2014, gauze squares sewn together with silk, 1500 x 2400cm   58
35. *Absence and Presence* 2014, gauze squares sewn together with silk, 1500 x 2400cm   60
36. *Energy 1* 2014, gauze squares sewn together with silk on chicken wire and acrylic, 1200 x 1200cm   61
37. *Energy 1* 2014, gauze squares sewn together with silk on chicken wire and acrylic, 1200 x 1200cm   62
38. *Chemotherapy* 2014, digital photograph   63
39. *Mercurochrome* 2014, digital photograph   63
40. Backlit prints installed in White Box Gallery, Griffith University, Gold Coast. 2015   64
41. *Shoe Covers* 2015, backlit print on radiology light box 75 x 60cm   64
42. *Vomit Bag* 2015, backlit print on radiology light box 60 x 75cm   65
43. *Theatre Towels* 2015, backlit print on radiology light box 75 x 60cm   66
44. *Isolation* 2014, surgical instruments mounted on patient gown, 1200 x 80cm   66
45. *Energy 2* 2015, light on organza, 1200 x 1200cm   68
46. *Absence and Presence* 2014, gauze squares sewn together with silk, 1500 x 2400cm   68
47. *Energy 1* 2014, gauze squares sewn together with silk on chicken wire and acrylic, 1200 x 1200cm   69
48. *Energy 1* 2014, gauze squares sewn together with silk on chicken wire and acrylic, 1200 x 1200cm   70
49. *Heart Starter, Mandala and Blade Holder* 2015, surgical instruments mounted on wood in situ in White Box Gallery, Griffith University, Gold Coast   71
50. *Absence and Presence* 2014, gauze squares sewn together with silk 1500 x 2400cm   72
51. *Unseen Gold* 2015, 1000-odd medicine cups   73

Acknowledgements

I am indebted to Associate Professor Donal Fitzpatrick for his continued support and insight. Thank you also to Dr Laini Burton and editor Evie Franzidis.

Thank you to family and friends for your encouragement over the last seven years.

I would also like to acknowledge nursing colleagues and patients from Hopewell Hospice, Gold Coast, for their contribution.

INTRODUCTION

Art and science are conventionally conceived of as opposing disciplines, representing radically different methodologies and practices. However, medicine is sometimes described as a combination of both art and science (Panda 2006). Within the medical sciences, the profession of nursing is characterised as a unique blend of the artistic principles of observation, interaction, and communication and the scientific principles of empiricism, analysis, and objective evaluation (Lumby 1991). Artistic values in nursing are represented by the subjective qualities of caring, empathy, and compassion. These combined attributes within nursing represent a set of active and operational intangibles that often defy rigorous definitive explanation or quantification. Nevertheless, I will discuss caring in more detail below, as it forms a major focal point of this research.

Caring is a highly complex human activity; as Judy Lumby notes, "It has been linked to love by many writers, and is regarded by Noddings as an ethical response to human need by both genders" (Lumby 1991, 7). Caring is not merely empathy, compassion, or warm feelings, but rather the external conveyance and communication of these feelings through a myriad of creative actions (Locsin 2001, 4). In nursing, caring involves the creative engagement of the senses in order to develop a meaningful understanding of a particular scenario. Thus, nursing can be seen as both an art and a science, and as such, a fine balance of these disciplines is needed in clinical practice. However, Watson (2002) suggests that in contemporary nursing there has been a depreciation of the caring aspect in contrast to its scientific development. Advances in medical technologies have provided nursing practitioners with new, effective, and fast-acting diagnostic tools. However, what was once noted through human contact and observation has been given over to machines, which has fundamentally altered the experiential nature of caring in nursing.

The depreciation of caring can be seen to coincide with the privileging of observation as a scientific practice, and vision as the primary sense through which knowledge is acquired. According to Plato, caring is an art or an expertise that is guided by the knowledge of the subject matter in question (Nordenfelt and Liss 2003, 15). Greek philosopher Hippocrates, revered as the founder of modern medicine, wrote extensively on the principles of observation. Kossolapow, Scoble, and Waller state that "The art of caring has been historically structured around a rational look or *the clinical eye*'"

(2003, 425). In *The Birth of the Clinic* (1973), Michel Foucault refers to such deep powers of observation as the 'medical gaze', which is a rigorous visual examination of its subject, an active and penetrating observation. As well as discussing the importance of observation, Florence Nightingale adds that 'reflection' is a crucial element of meaningful practice in her *Notes on Nursing*. Rob van der Peet cites Nightingale as writing:

> "Reflection needs training as much as observation. Observation tells us the fact; reflection the meaning of the fact." It is interesting to note that Nightingale's injunction at the end of the nineteenth century to think about what is being observed and act on this is now, a century later, a central concept in the notion of the reflective practitioner being adopted in nursing under the influences of writers such as Schon. (van der Peet 1995, 47)

In contemporary nursing science, the definition of caring that is grounded in both theory and empirical findings is framed as "a nurturing way of relating to a valued other towards whom one feels a personal sense of commitment and responsibility" (Watson 2002, 203). Certain 'carative factors' that are essential within nursing science include the altruistic values of empathy and compassion, sensitivity to self and others, the instillation of faith-hope, and the development of helping-trust relationships (Watson 2002). It is also essential to treat people as individuals. Carl G. Jung (1961, 153) stated, "To my mind, in dealing with individuals, only individual understanding will do. We need a different language for every patient." Kossolapow et al. (2003, 425) provide a more contemporary vision of care, stating that "the therapeutic activity of caring in its practical declination brings about the issue of subjectivity, relationship, emotions and their possible depictions, and the mirroring of identity profiles of the various actors involved in the theatre of caring". Caring can thus be seen as a complex interpersonal experience requiring a sensory engagement beyond that of the solely visual. This understanding of caring can be likened to the aesthetic experience, which Susan Buck-Morss (1992, 6) describes as a "form of cognition achieved through taste, touch, hearing, seeing and smell".

The interpersonal experience of caring associated with nursing is the demonstrated act of "authentic presence" that creates a sense of connectedness, resulting in a positive experience for both nurse and patient. Communicating authentic presence is based on the nurse actually being what he or she seems to be. This authentic presence or being genuine, honest, and without front is what psychotherapist Carl Rogers describes as congruence (Gendlin 1959). This ability to be open with the feelings and attitudes that are within at any given moment is critical in the interpersonal nurse–patient relationship (Watson 1985, 26). As academic and nursing theorist Jean Watson states, "Human care can begin when the nurse enters into the life space of the phenomenal field of the other" (Watson quoted in Kuhse 1997, 149).

The ideas of 'authentic' experience and the 'phenomenal field' can be equated with Walter Benjamin's analysis of 'aura'. Benjamin describes aura as follows: "If while resting on a summer afternoon, you follow with your eyes a mountain range on the horizon or a branch, which casts its shadow over you, you experience the aura of those mountains, of that branch" (Benjamin 1936, 5). The condition of the direct experience of the object in Benjamin's concept of the 'aura' is predicated on a particular understanding of aesthetics. Contemporary understandings of aesthetics are most often associated with ideas of vision and beauty, but Benjamin's usage relates more to the totality of human sense perception, which makes his idea of 'aura' a useful tool in elucidating the interpersonal experience of caring in the context of nursing (Benjamin 1936).

Some nursing academics have labelled Watson as "a navel gazer and skeptic" (Kuhse 1997, 149), and theorist Alan Sokai discredits and challenges her perspective in *Beyond the Hoax: Science, Philosophy and Culture* (Sokai 2008, 446). However, her observations resonate with my own extensive experience as a registered nurse, particularly the time I spent in palliative care over the last nine years of my nursing career.

During my active working life, I observed advances in medicine and the influence and resultant transformation of nursing's role towards a more exclusive scientific approach.

This paradigm shift has not been without cost to those elusive qualities previously identified as some of the hallmarks of the nursing profession. In turn, this prompted my research, which is framed around the following question: In what ways can the disciplines of nursing and fine art inform each other in relation to the emotional and material circumstances of the medical environment?

As this research operates within an interdisciplinary space between art and nursing, I will begin this exegesis by outlining a brief historical overview of the interrelationship between nursing and the arts. Next, I will explore the research question in its significance and importance. Thereafter, I will present a critical reading of selected artists' work that highlights some of the key issues of this research.

Finally, I will examine my own studio practice and expound on the personal contribution that my research brings to the interpersonal encounter between nurse and patient. This research is directly relevant to the nursing industry through its unpacking and examining of the power and efficacy of the subjective qualities of the nursing experience. Through its deployment of studio experiments, it will bring nursing practice into the arena of the visual through a celebration and acknowledgement of the shared presence of nurse and patient.

CHAPTER 1: NURSING AND THE VISUAL ARTS

In this chapter, I will give a brief overview of the nurse as interpreted through the visual arts. The visual arts and nursing share a complex, multifaceted history. The figure of the nurse has been represented since approximately 20,000 BC (Donohue 1985, 25). Because nursing has historically been perceived as a social necessity rather than a legitimate profession, its social status has been confined to the lower ranks of service. As one source notes, "In primitive times for example she was a slave, and in the civilised era, a domestic. Over-looked in the plans of the legislators, and forgotten in the curricula of pedagogues, she was left without protection and remained without education" (Robinson quoted in Donohue 1985, 1). Importantly, Victor Robinson notes that while "the untrained nurse is as old as the human race, the trained nurse is a relatively new concept, emerging with Florence Nightingale in 1860" (Robinson quoted in Donohue 1985, 1).

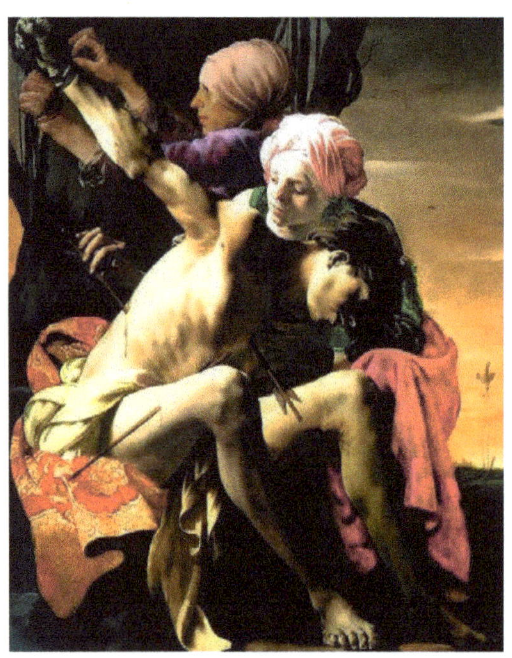

Figure 1 Hendrick Terbruggen
St. Sebastian Attended by St. Irene

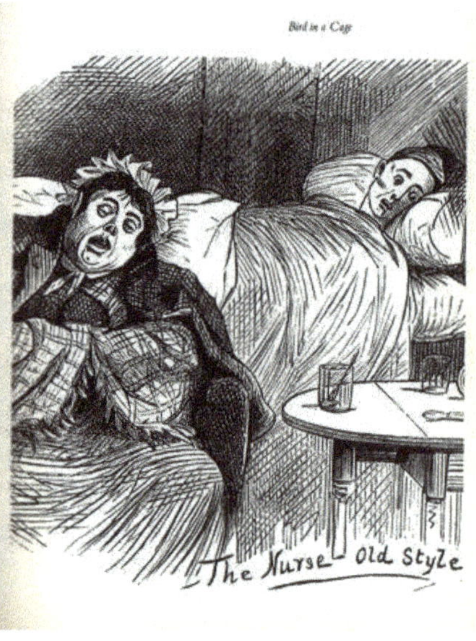

Figure 2 Anonymous
The Old Style Nurse

Not only has nursing long been associated with women and women's work through the ages, but it has also operated beyond this gendered stereotype as an index of the place and status of women more broadly in society (Hudson-Jones 1988, 6). This is substantiated by the diversity of the historical representations of the nurse, in which the nurse is aligned with diametrically opposing concepts such as mother and seductress, healing saint and prostitute (see figures 1 and 2). Nursing still carries with it the connotations of its etymological foundation to give nourishment, and its long association with women and women's work seems to characterise it as a natural requirement of life rather than as part of a socio-economic system. This location of nursing within the domain of the feminine has confined it to an ill-defined zone of marginal work and remuneration (Lumby 1991).

Representations of the nurse are accordingly paradoxical and contradictory as they attempt to capture an image that both attracts and repels. Visual art has been significant in tracing the genesis and evolving practice of nursing through images. The nurse has functioned as a metaphor for values associated with women, and the tensions in nursing today reflect historical and contemporary conflicts about women's role in society, the workplace, and societal values.[1] Historical representations of the nurse help us understand the stereotypical labels that have been placed on the contemporary nurse. Images of the professional nurse are limited, which may be due to the many duties of a nurse that are considered mundane and boring in contrast to the heroic feats of a doctor or surgeon (Lumby 1991), as seen in Thomas Eakins's famous painting *The Agnew Clinic* (figure 3).

---

[1] Nursing is recognised as a female-dominated industry, and it has traditionally been a feminised role; approximately 10% of nurses working within Australian Healthcare today are male (Australian Bureau of Statistics 2013).

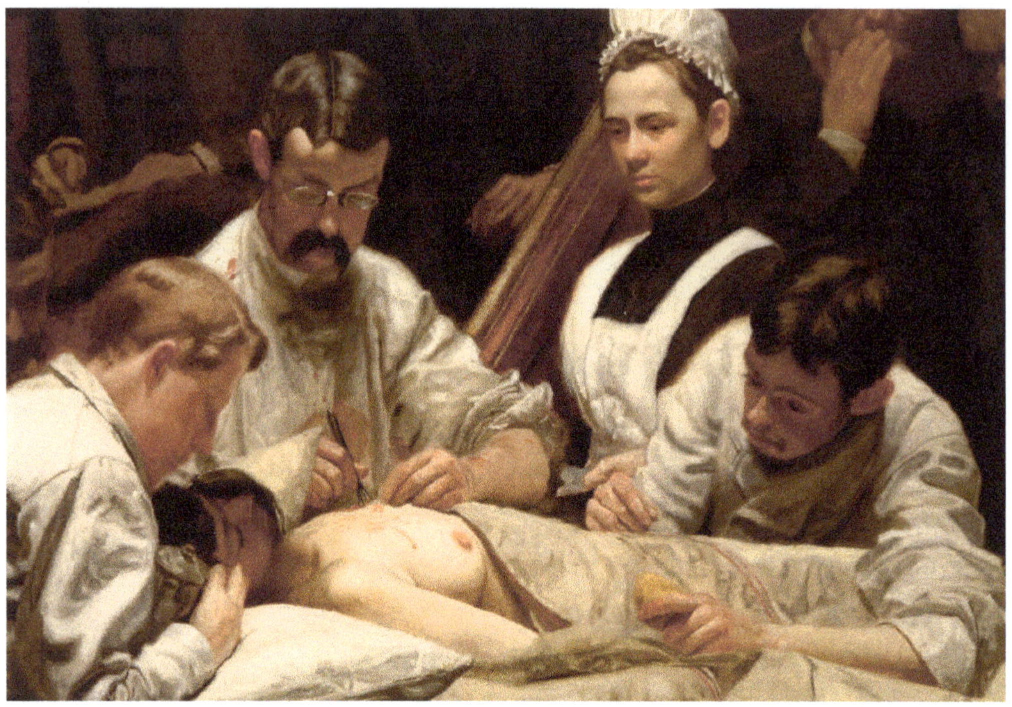

Figure 3 Thomas Eakins *The Agnew Clinic* (detail)

For the sick, who are human beings at their most vulnerable, the image of a nurse can oscillate between positive and negative, an angel and a witch, comfort and pain. Disease, personality, and pain influence this image, as the patient's sense of self is often shattered during illness. As Jean Rousselot (1967, 8) states, "Sickness and suffering are the potent acids that penetrate the human heart and lay bare its most secret corners." By its nature, nursing operates on this deeply intimate level. This intimacy allows the nurse to violate the usual social taboos by seeing and touching patients' bodies. In turn, this has given rise to eroticised images (figures 4 and 5) of the nurse as someone outside the conventions of human behaviour and yet deeply enmeshed in the value systems that we identify as most human; namely, the care and consideration of others.

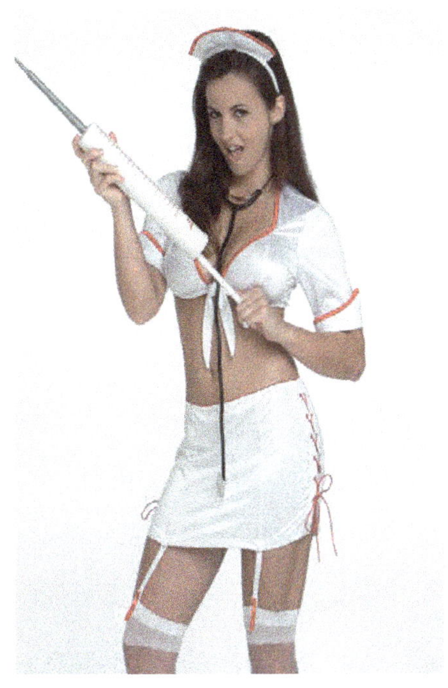

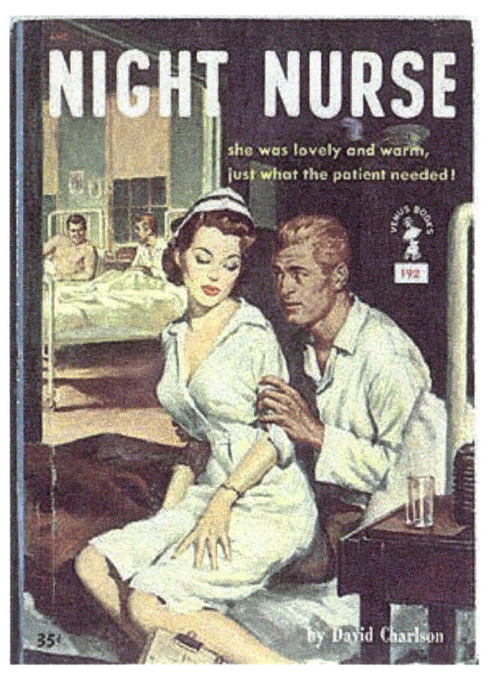

Figure 4 Novelty Nurse Costume   **Figure 5** Book cover, 1950s

Multiple layers of meaning operate within the concept of the 'nurse' which differ depending on the situation and state of the patient. However, the expert nurse can detect a patient's response to his/her image and respond appropriately. As Benner states:

> When an individual becomes a master of his or her cultures or practices, or a professional practice within it, he or she no longer tries to do what one normally does, but rather responds out of a fund of experiences in the culture and in the specialised practice. This requires having enough experience to give up following the rules and maxims dictating what anyone should do, and instead acting upon the intuition that results from a life in which talent and sensibility have allowed learning from the experience of satisfaction and regret in similar situations. (Benner quoted in Rolfe 1997, 94)

Much of accumulated knowledge gained by nurses cannot be easily explained or put into words. Benner refers to nursing actions as the 'intuitive grasp' of a process by which the nurse just seems to know the right thing to do in any given situation. Thus, as Rolfe concludes:

> The expert nurse is therefore a reflective practitioner who processes his/her experiences through reflection-on-action into personal knowledge and paradigm cases, and then smoothly and unconsciously translates that knowledge into practice, displaying an intuitive grasp of whatever situation he/she finds herself in. (Rolfe, 1997, 95)

This creative process is the taking, absorbing, and feeling of many experiences from the past and the blending of them with the occasions that present themselves in the moment to influence future experiences. According to Alfred Whitehead's philosophy, momentarily developing experiences are the basic building blocks of all reality. While we exist one experience at a time, our bodies exist many experiences at a time (Society for the Study of Process Philosophy n.d.). Nowhere is this truer than in nursing practice.

When nurse and patient meet as interactive beings within the medical space, the nurse is exposed to the direct suffering and vulnerability of the patient; here, the core values of caring, empathy, and compassion are paramount. In the next chapter, I will explore the research question and how my research aims to elucidate these values.

CHAPTER 2: EXPLORING THE RESEARCH QUESTION

As stated in the introduction, this research was framed around the following question: In what ways can the disciplines of nursing and fine art inform each other in relation to the emotional and material circumstances of the medical environment? Nursing is a physical business and nurses use their bodies, especially their hands, as the primary tool in their work. While the labour-intensive aspects of nursing remain fundamental to the role, they are somewhat misunderstood and unread. As such, in the works produced during the early stages of this research, I depicted nurses in a representational manner to draw viewers' attention to the physical work of nursing.

However, as my research progressed, I became more interested in the spaces in which private dialogues occur between nurse and patient, which is both secret and silent and, in essence, invisible. Specifically, I became interested in examining the spaces within which medicine and healthcare take place, the particularity of the function and operation of silence within these spaces, and its effect on both the patient and the nurse. The silence within the medical environment is at odds with the characteristics of a workplace of hard physical labour. While this silence evokes abstract notions of reverence, it is in actuality motivated by fear. The body is an unwelcome guest; a reminder of unknown danger and mortality. For these and other reasons, we can evaluate the separation of practices and the operation of hierarchies that are based on their distance from the 'body as person' and any direct engagement with the 'body as work'.

Nursing operates in a materially and emotionally charged environment, with nurses present at some of life's monumental occasions: the joy and pain of childbirth; the experience of well-being and recovery after illness; and the pain and helplessness of death. This research project unpacks and examines the power and efficacy of the subjective qualities of the professional nursing experience and brings these phenomena into the arena of the visual arts where, to date, there has been limited and muted representation. As Lumby states, "Their silence is evident in the absence of texts, paintings and research by women. Science has enforced this silence by devaluing the everyday, the self understanding, the subjective knowledge that women have and develop so well" (1991, 8). Tracing the shifting role and iconography of the nurse opens up and exposes the complexity of this figure for critical analysis.

Illness itself is intangible and functions as an often contradictory experience, sometimes at odds with our sensory bodily perception; yet, it exposes the absolute materiality and transitory vulnerability of the body. We have ample examples of horror and the gaping expression of quantitative pain, but the image of illness itself is seemingly so subtle as to defy visual description. These considerations led me to the active role and contribution of the mute everyday objects of the medical environment to determine the perception and values of medicalised space and their capacity to both trigger and capture the passing of the elusive phenomenon of illness.

Despite the increasingly technological nature of the medical environment, the fundamental work of nursing has remained consistent because patient's basic human needs are unchanging. Therefore, the guiding principle in nursing is care of the physical body, and a deep concern with the patient as a holistic being. Within this complex working space, defined as it is by pain and discomfort, the nurse is by association linked with the numerous industrial implements and devices of the medical environment characterised by negative psychological connotations, such as needles, forceps, and bedpans, to name but a few (figures 6 and 7).

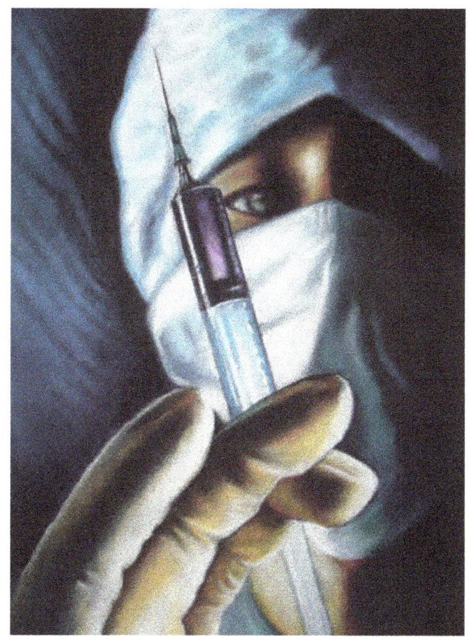

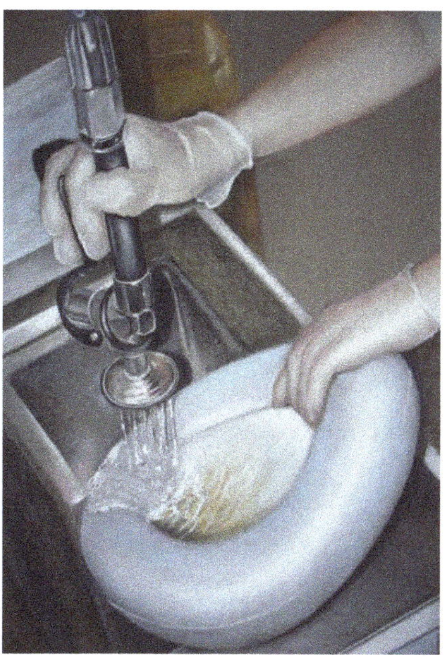

Figure 6 Hazel Cope *This Will Hurt!*   **Figure 7** Hazel Cope *Voided 500mls*

These types of everyday medical industrial objects that are ubiquitous in the medical and
hospital environment are most commonly viewed by patients with apprehension or
embarrassment because they are associated with the transgression of the patient's body.
For a patient, objects in the medical environment can function at an emotive level,
inducing fear and indignation as they can trigger a memory that may reconstruct an
unpleasant experience. The objects assigned to the patient in the context of care expose
the abject nature of the body—excreta, wounds, and blood. Those objects associated with
abjection in the medical arena such as catheter and stoma bags can be viewed by the
patient with resentment and are a constant reminder of the limitations of their physical
self. These attributes ascribed to the paraphernalia of applied medicine are emotionally
encoded through the patients' conflation of the objects with their function.

However, the objects themselves are benign; it is their context that is imbued with
negative associations. Medical professionals use these objects and devices to provide
care. However, nurses often inflict pain by using needles to administer pain relief or
antibiotics. Thus, paradoxically, the nurse inflicts pain through objects aimed to relieve
pain and promote health. I have been drawn to the role of the materials of the medical

environment because they capture the often-elusive qualities that exist within the special theatre of illness and the nursing experience.

My research project examines the changing aesthetic of these medical utilitarian objects and explores their re-coding from industrial purpose into works of art through my deployment of the artistic processes of repetition and unfamiliar placement. I aim to explore and valorise the subtle phenomena present in the interconnection and relationship between nurse and patient and to bring its quality and feeling into a visible form. The research seeks to contribute a qualitative dimension of nursing experience and practice that is not for the purposes of instruction or for the glorification and heroism of medicine most commonly represented for the male practitioner (as seen in the Eakins painting illustrated earlier). In the next chapter, I will consider the changes that have taken place in contemporary nursing due to technological advances as well as time pressures.

CHAPTER 3: TIME AND TECHNOLOGY

In this chapter, I will discuss the factors that have contributed to the changes seen in the interrelationships between nurses and patients in contemporary health care. While caring for patients, nurses get to know them and are able to determine their individual wishes and concerns, as well as provide comfort and compassion to them. This quality of care is dependent on human interactions between nurse and patient, which in turn requires time. One of the greatest threats to caring in nursing practice today is that less time is available for nurses to engage with their patients due to increased paperwork, advances in technology, and downsizing (Cluff and Binstock 2001, 128). Frank Davidoff suggests that the growing trend towards alternative medicine within Western society can be partly explained by the fact that its practitioners have more time to give to patients and provide a more holistic approach to care (quoted in Cluff and Binstock 2001, 129).

The consistent rise in administrative responsibilities over the last ten years is preventing nurses from spending time with their patients ("Nurses 'Drowning in a Sea of Paperwork'" 2013). Therefore, the authentic one-on-one experience of nurses and patients is in decline. While good documentation is vital in nursing, the increase in litigation, accreditation, and economic targets has caused vast swathes of unnecessary paperwork. In a recent survey conducted by the Royal College of Nursing in the UK, it was found that 17.3% of a registered nurse's time is spent undertaking non-essential paperwork such as filing and photocopying ("Nurses 'Drowning in a Sea of Paperwork'" 2013). The danger is that this is undermining nurses' ability to care for patients, which is crucial in maintaining the authentic interpersonal experience of care. Watson notes,

> At a time when nursing is declining and its survival threatened, nursing satisfaction is enhanced when caring is able to be practiced. When caring is not present in nursing practices or settings, research indicates that nurses become depressed, robotic, hardened, oblivious, and worn down. (Watson 2002, 16–17)

Another issue that contributes to the diminution of the authentic caring experience is the increasing dynamic of technology. The hard data supplied by sophisticated technological devices in some areas of nursing often serve as the final guide on how to treat a patient. This is problematic as these devices supply so much precise numerical information that less attention is paid to what patients feel and say about their illness (Swanbrow 1995). Here the patient's body is a machine under the control of the nurse, and there is a danger of a lack of human interconnectedness. Thus, machines and technology can be seen as a barrier to the interpersonal experience of nursing, Dr. John Howell maintains that with an overuse of technology, health professionals are becoming better scientists but poorer healers, and a step back from the current trend is needed (Swanbrow 1995). This trend is seen in some countries such as Japan and the USA, which regard technology as a solution to aging populations and nurse shortages. In Japan, robot nurses such as 'Actroid F' have been designed to provide companionship to the aged. These robot nurses are able to mimic facial expressions and repeat rudimentary sentences, yet they are devoid of all human emotion and authentic engagement (Dubroff 2010). In the USA, robots visit patients, dispense medicines and transport materials such as food, linen and X-rays throughout hospitals (Dubroff 2010). Although such machines are useful in some aspects of care, such as lifting patients and delivering linen, philosopher Slavoj Žižek (1997, 130–31) warns against the uncritical celebration, or fearful rejection, of new technologies. Instead, he advocates that we actively engage with them while at the same time maintaining a critical distance, so that we remain aware of exactly what we are losing and gaining in moments of technological transition.

The increase of diagnostic tools and lifesaving technology has extended both the length and quality of life for people. However, Dianne Swanbrow questions whether machines are getting in the way of one of medicine's major goals—easing the suffering of sick people (Swanbrow 1995). Nurses are increasingly observing machines rather than patients. Thus, the full sensory involvement of the interpersonal relationship between nurse and patient is in danger of being lost, as vision is privileged over all other senses.

As caring is an art, it needs to continually push boundaries and be redefined. Thus, the use of new technologies could be construed as a new form of caring, and patients expect nurses to be proficient in using new technology. However, technological competence alone does not result in caring. The qualities of empathy, kindness, compassion, and open communication with patients are indispensable in all aspects of nursing care. As Rozzano Locsin articulates, "Nurses who are expert in communicating caring effectively go *to* the patient *through* the technology, not stopping with attending to tubes and monitors, but first connecting with the patient through authentic presence" (2001, 8, original emphasis). Buck-Morss's explanation of Benjamin's concerns about the cultural impact of technology is highly relevant here. Buck-Morss claims that through his recommendation to politicise art, Benjamin is demanding that art should attempt to "*undo* the alienation of the corporeal sensorium, to restore the *instinctual power of the human bodily senses for the sake of humanity's self preservation,* and to do this, not by avoiding the new technologies, but by *passing through* them" (Buck-Morss 1992, 5, original emphasis). Technological advancement can therefore be seen to pose a possible threat to both the authentic interpersonal caring experience in nursing and art, a threat that is crucially linked to the diminution of the aesthetic experience.

With the advancements in technology, working as a nurse in critical areas such as intensive care can be both challenging and exciting, as opposed to palliative care or geriatric nursing, which is a permanent reminder of the less appealing and denied values of the human. The hierarchical system of nursing affords the nurses who work in clean areas with machines or in teaching or managerial positions a higher status, even though they have no direct association with the patient's body. This is reflected both in the status of the nursing profession and in the wages paid.

With the increase in imaging technologies and diagnostics, there has been an accelerated reliance on machines and visual data in understanding both the body and those mental, emotional, and spiritual elements that remain hidden and unseen. In her book *Body Criticism: Imaging the Unseen in Enlightenment Art and Medicine* (1997), Barbara Maria Stafford substantiates how vital visual culture has been in the understanding of the human body throughout history. Many cultures have relied upon the procedures of dissection, marking, and sensing, to name but a few, and translated these to the visual to understand the human being.

The arts are often dismissed as only a therapeutic modality; for example, Art and Diversional Therapy. However, the visual in medicine as both a therapeutic and technological assistant within diagnosis and education is often underappreciated in the science-dominated professions. This presents a contradiction: the marginalisation of the attributes of the arts within the sciences and a concurrent dependency upon the development and proliferation of numerous imaging systems. Often unrecognised for their critical evaluation and veracity, the visual arts and design are crucial to the operation of medicine and patient care. There is a gaping epistemological space that exists between art and science imaging and how images have served one and the other in vastly different ways. My studio research aims to bridge that gap by making visible the values of empathy, compassion, and caring in nursing practice. I will now turn to a discussion of the 'everyday' in both nursing and art so as to contextualise the visual art outcomes of this research.

CHAPTER 4: THE 'EVERDAY' OF NURSING AND ART

In this chapter, I examine the 'everyday' of both the nurse–patient experience and the 'everyday' as it pertains to the visual arts. The 'everyday' is described as those objects and commonplaces that are trivial, ordinary, boring and repetitive, those nonevents that make up the mundane aspects of everyday life ("Everyday" 2015). Like our bodies, commonplace objects share the physicality of our world and they are understood to have an independent physicality, and be substances in their own right, being both optical and perceptual phenomena that contain their own essence and energy (Pearce 1994). Objects convey their own unique code and have the dynamic mnemonic capacity to trigger memories and emotions. In a way, objects define us and our lives, be they designer clothes, furniture, jewelry, or an individually designed wheelchair. They influence the very way we relate to each other, how we look at each other, whether we will stand or sit, where we will eat, and how we live in our everyday lives (Sudjic 2008). While the hospital space is 'everyday' for the nurse, it is not a commonplace but an unusual situation for those in care and, for the most part, temporary, even for those at the end of life; therefore, it is not 'everyday' for patients.

The concept of the medical patient is one of intense displacement away from familiarity, comfort, and loved ones. The sick patient is not only vulnerable in relation to the direct casualty of their illness but also to the concomitant challenge to their autonomy and subordination of a sense of self. Most nurses are witness to the immediate needs and the suffering of others as well as the mortality of human beings. The nursing experience is associated 'as presence' at moments of intense personal emotion and grief and at the cessation of life. Furthermore, the nurse becomes aware of the depth dimension of the body as living flesh in the ordinary care encounter behind the screens, while being totally present in the moment.

Caring for the diseased body and vulnerable self is the domain of nursing, with direct care of the body described as 'dirty work' through the cleaning up of bodily excreta, faeces, urine, sputum, blood, and vomit (Lawler 2006, 4). This area of nursing where the nurse is closest to the patient's abject body is coded within a derogatory context and assigned to the lowest status of nursing. According to Holmes et al. (quoted in Wolf 2013, 56), the unclean aspect of nursing and how it affects nurses is seldom critically examined in academic literature.

Care of the body is privatised and not available for public perusal. This is because many nursing duties transgress 'normal' social boundaries and can be embarrassing, nauseating, and considered dirty or sexual. The performance, execution, and skill of nursing duties can be measured; for example, dressing a fungating, foul-smelling tumour. However, the way or 'the manner' in which these duties are carried out cannot be measured and is in the domain of feeling. In handling a patient, a nurse can touch gently or roughly, be kind with words or abrupt. The way in which the nurse carries out his or her duties is an outward manifestation of their inner qualities of compassion, or lack thereof. Understanding that the patient is not just an objectified body contributes to an authentic interpersonal connection between nurse and patient. The experienced nurse practitioner performs their duties with the awareness that the patient is an embodied being. When this happens, the patient is able to sense that they are valued as a human. For a nurse to have this awareness and act upon it with intelligence and creativity in a myriad of nursing situations also requires a complex interpersonal experience and sensory engagement beyond that of the solely visual.

Nurses confront the abject body as part of their daily work and learn to reject their own sensibilities to maintain professional behaviour (Holmes quoted in Wolf 2013, 56). In dealing with abjection, nurses use tolerance, humour, peer support, and resilience. In her book *Exploring Nursing Rituals: Joining Art and Science,* Zane Robinson Wolf explores the rituals in nursing such as bathing that help to maintain human dignity and respect when dealing with the abject body (Wolf 2013). This is especially significant when nurses continue their care of a patient's body after death. Nurses care for the post-mortem patient in a variety of settings—a patient's home, accident and emergency departments' intensive care, and palliative care wards. Here, the abject body and the mystery of death and suffering, the sacred and the profane, become combined elements in the nurse's tasks.

The person is still acknowledged as 'being present' when nurses bathe their dead bodies, remove medical devices from them, and prepare their bodies for viewing. However, nursing practice is in essence about people's experiences of embodied existence, specifically at those times when the body is dysfunctional. Jocalyn Lawler explores this in her book *Behind the Screens: Nursing, Somology, and the Problem of the Body* (2006). This book seeks to explicate the highly private work and socially unacceptable aspects of nursing that are rarely discussed. It reveals the difficulties that nurses experience in their care of the patient's bodies and explores topics such as dirty work, excreta and genitalia (Lawler 2006).

The 'everyday' experience of work in palliative care nursing is significant and often extraordinary, as nurses not only attend to patient care, write care plans, and reports but also assist patients and their families to partake in final conversations, special family gatherings, and last meals together. Pain, administration of pain relief, loss of consciousness, and confusion often interject these special times, together with doctors' visits and the numerous responsibilities of nursing and ancillary staff. These are the 'everyday' experiences of a palliative care ward. However, many patients have no relatives and the nurse can become a confidante and a trusted friend. The elusive qualities of the caring experience are high in palliative care and are self-evident to those who are being cared for as they speak of nursing in artistic terms: "the 'gentleness' of the touch, the 'sensitivity' of the handling, the 'empathy' of the listening" (Lumby 1991, 28). The ephemeral is palpable in the dying process, and the nurse is a grounding 'presence'.

The everyday space in these settings can change quickly, as a patient's condition can worsen within hours. At these times, the nurse is acutely observant and on high alert to attend to the changing needs of patients and families, as emotions can oscillate between intense anxiety and exquisite pleasure. The experienced nurse knows how to listen, communicate, and accept the circumstances without prejudice and judgment, as responses to grief are individualistic. This attitude of the nurse is an expression of phenomenology, a way of thinking introduced by Maurice Merleau-Ponty in 1945 that considers experience in a holistic way rather than separating the mind from the body, as in Cartesian thought ([1945] 1962). In nursing, a phenomenological approach focuses on the importance of understanding a patient's lived experience as pertaining to him/her personally, rather than merely the given facts of the illness a patient may be facing (Balls 2009). Phenomenology is now used as a qualitative research methodology to understand a patient's meaning of a particular situation and is also incorporated as experiential training for undergraduate nurses (Balls 2009).

Asking questions, being aware of nonverbal communication and mannerisms, and perceiving a patient's feelings and emotions to their current situation without prejudice and judgment are part of the interpretative phenomenological attitude that is fundamental to palliative care nursing. As Lawler states: "For nurses, the clinical gaze is extended from external features of the patient's body to the private thoughts, feelings and everyday lives of patients in the quest to find the patient's authentic self" (Lawler quoted in Lupton 2008, 124). Working with this phenomenological attitude while performing nursing duties, such as wound care, measuring, and administering dangerous drugs, exemplifies the intertwining nature of both the subjective and objective experience of the nurse.

The 'everyday' has been the subject of much visual art over the last century. For the 11th Biennale of Sydney themed 'Everyday', curator Jonathan Watkins chose works that sought to go beyond the common object to bring attention to the actuality and unseen aspects of our lives, as epitomised in the work of Germaine Koh *Knitwork* (figure 8).

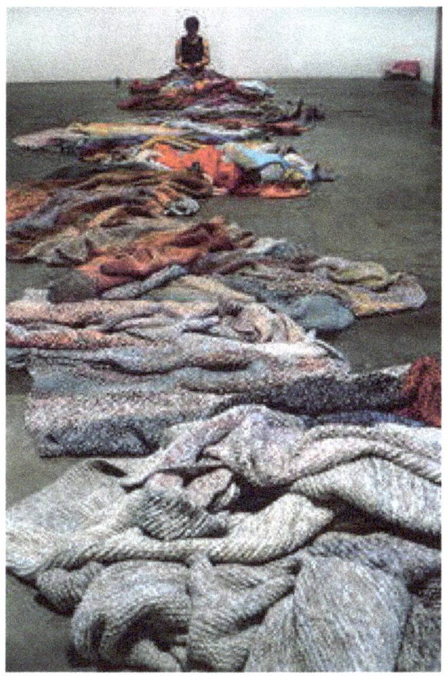

Figure 8 Germaine Koh *Knitwork*

In this work, Koh unravels unwanted knitwear such as scarves and jumpers and re-knits the spun thread into a single growing object, which is placed in the gallery space. This has been an ongoing work since 1992. The absence of a point of completion emphasises the grace of the continuous present and is a visual record of the passage of time (Watkins 1998, 140). Koh states: "the work will be completed when I cease to be" (Koh 2005).

In her review of Stephen Johnstone's anthology *The Everyday* (2008), Jennifer Dyer refers to French philosopher Simone Weil's definition of attention as a contemplative practice with an unbiased/unpossessive openness to the other (Dyer 2009). The attention to the everyday was first realised by Marcel Duchamp when he made this a deliberate and conscious discovery with his work *Fountain* (1917). This work and the famous furor surrounding its reception and rejection by the Society of the Independent Artists in New York were outlined in great detail by Thierry de Duve, who characterised the jury's rejection of the work *Fountain*, an ordinary urinal, on the grounds that it was not a product made by the artist and not an original work (de Duve quoted in Formis 2004). Indeed, de Duve's thesis stipulates that to have accepted this object as a work of art would have invalidated the very understanding of what a work of art was, and that this act of subversion was exactly what the object *Fountain* achieved (Formis, 2004, 249–50).

However, Barbara Formis has argued that rather than being a pure piece of subversion, *Fountain* offered a more exquisite manifestation of the essence of art, in revealing what she terms the ontological site of the work. She points out that the readymade dramatically underscored the truth that all art is always, at an ontological level, a readymade. For example, paintings always require all forms of industrial manufacture—brushes, tubes of paint, canvas, stretchers, etc.—in order to exist. The readymade in this context opens up an ambiguous space within the world of art. As Formis writes:

> On the one hand, the readymade reveals an important truth: works of art need ordinary objects in order to exist, art lies inevitably within a bedrock of no-art; on the other hand, this first truth automatically implies a reciprocal truth: works of art do not necessarily have more value than ordinary objects. (Formis 2004, 250)

This chapter has considered the concept of the 'everyday' as it pertains to nursing and visual art. The next chapter will examine the practice of several visual artists whose work has explored similar themes to my own.

CHAPTER 5: CONTEXTUAL REVIEW

In this chapter, I will discuss the work of certain artists whose work is linked to the thematic concerns of my research. Robert Pope and Rebecca Horn attempt to address the visceral reality of illness through their response to the experience of their hospitalisations. Richard Prince, William Kentridge, Michael Elmgreen, and Ingar Dragset investigate the shifting visual relations present in the medical environment. The analysis of chosen images highlights some of the issues of this research and draws out elements of the theoretical concerns.

Robert Pope

Pope's depictions of the journey of a patient expose the vulnerability, pain, and isolation that are associated with cancer, chemotherapy, and its associated treatments. Over a decade-long personal ordeal, Pope painted ninety-six life-size canvases, which were highly descriptive yet minimalist works of medical testing, doctors, and hospital surroundings. Many of his works embody the personal suffering associated with illness and communicate the human aspect of disease and hospitalisation in a direct and emotional way. He dramatically illustrates the cold and dehumanising experiences of diagnosis and treatment within contemporary healthcare (figure 9).

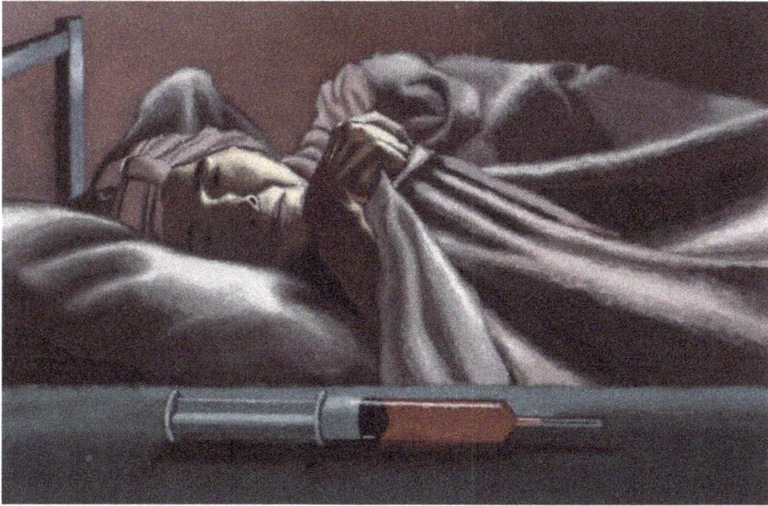

Figure 9 Robert Pope *Chemotherapy*

Some of his paintings vividly convey close human contacts and evoke love, strength, and the hope of healing as in *Sparrow* (1989, figure 10). As many of his works are self-portraits, they convey the contradictory nature of the patient's experience as both ill body and vigorous subject or person. In the late 1980s, Pope made seminar presentations on his artistic works to young medical students in order to convey his lived experiences and observations of illness. His interest was to listen to individual responses to his paintings; he believed that an artwork was only complete when the work and the person perceiving it came together because everyone has a unique life and thus a unique perception (Murray 1995, 111).

Doctors have used Pope's work to help medical students understand what it feels like to be a patient. By viewing the works, they gain an insight into how a patient is really feeling. His life-size paintings overwhelm the viewer and trigger feelings of empathy and compassion. Furthermore, his book *Illness and Healing* (Pope 2004) has become widely used as part of the medical humanities programs in his native Canada to engender compassion and understanding in medical students.

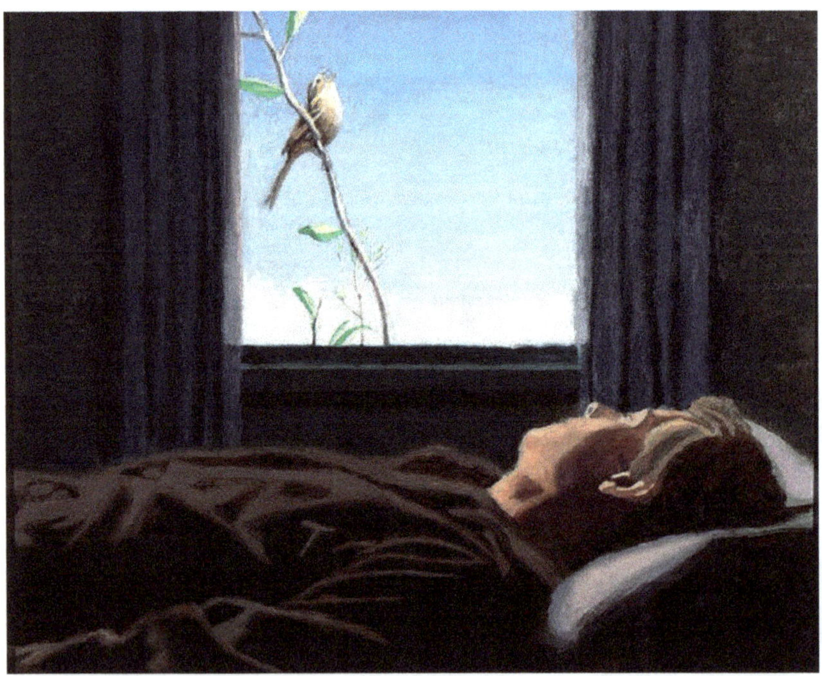

Figure 10 Robert Pope *Sparrow*

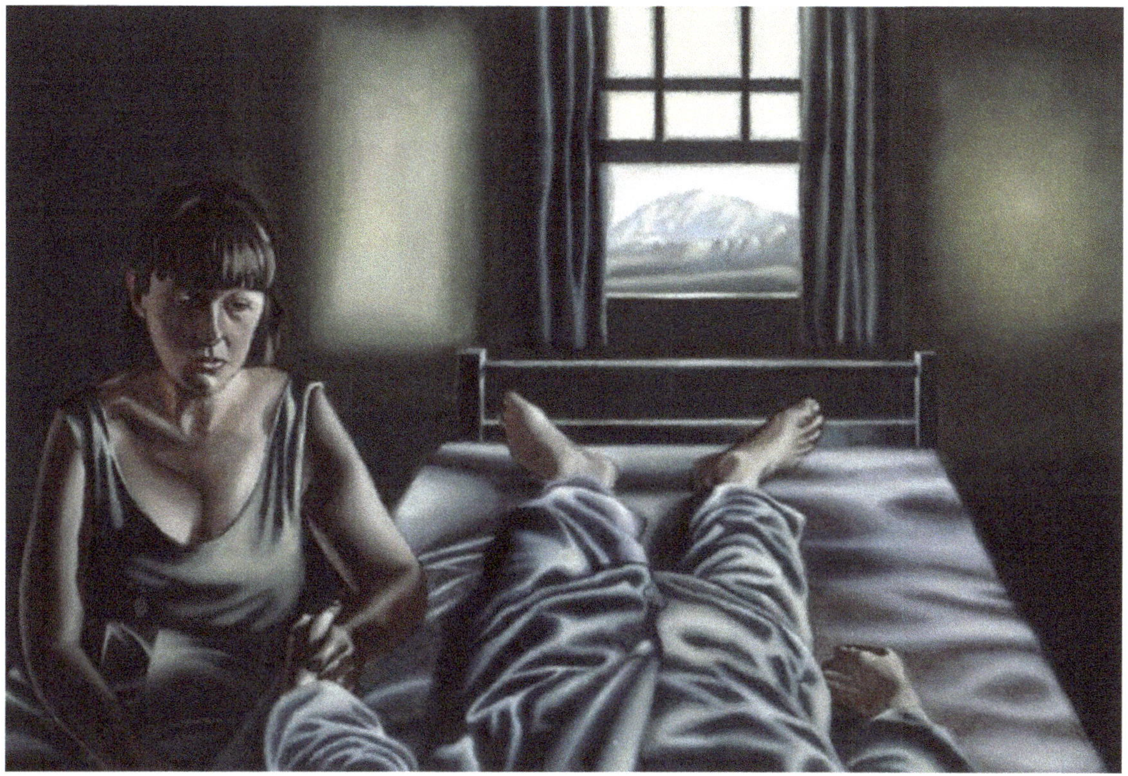

Figure 11 Robert Pope *Mountain*

Many of Pope's paintings show his body and feet viewed from his position on the bed, as well as the world beyond. The viewpoint contained in *Mountain* (1990, figure 11) is typical of a patient's field of vision. The work shows the patient in fresh pajamas and in a relaxed position after being washed and cleaned by the nurse. This is the state in which visitors often encounter long-term hospital patients.

The eponymous mountain depicted in the distance in *Mountain* is a metaphor not only for Pope's illness and the enormous challenge it presents, but also a symbol of hope and the healing power of nature, which is a common theme in Pope's work. The mountain can also stand for wildness or the uncontrolled, both as a form of nostalgia for a previous wellness and an elusive desire for something beyond the heavily controlled environment of the hospital. Although illness is a singular experience, Pope shows that it involves others and can be a time when bonds between loved family members and close friends are experienced in previously unfelt ways. This work reveals the enormous value and significance of these relationships that endure through all the ups and downs of sickness and hospitalisation. It is not just the patient who undergoes a perplexing range of emotions and responses but also their immediate family and friends.

However, this painting is also a portrayal of the loss of independence and the reliance on others that is emblematic of our human interconnectedness. Nursing is one of the situations that embodies our interdependence and, in a literal sense, is emblematic of what Merleau-Ponty calls our inter-subjectivity (Merleau-Ponty quoted in Krysl 2012, 2). As Drew Leder states: "The full reality of this sensible world arises not simply from the power of sight, or any such mode, but from the mutual reference and intertwining of all forms of perception" (Leder 1990, 211).

This painting not only captures the support of the loved one but also the anxiety and awkward silence that can accompany visiting a loved one; the sweaty palms and the sense of helplessness. Fear and concern are seen in the woman's face as deeply personal vulnerabilities and fears surface ranging from the anger of failed medical treatment to the loss of a loved family member and the struggle when facing mortality.

Rebecca Horn

Hospitalised in a sanatorium for over a year with a chest complaint, Rebecca Horn experienced the isolation and challenges associated with severe illness. Being confined in a hospital bed, her response to this experience was to explore ideas of touch and sensation. This was done by making balsa wood fingers to extend her body from the hospital bed. *Finger Gloves* (1972, figure 12) was one of Horn's earliest performance works and displays how the balsa wood fingers clumsily search out space and objects and yet have no functionality.

They depict the awkwardness and changed perception experienced by those undergoing an illness. In many cases, illness does not have outward signs of physical difference. Wearing the gloves, Horn is able to touch objects at a distance, giving her the illusion in her mind that she is actually touching the objects she is viewing. Her exploration to reach out is maintained throughout her performance piece, validating her ability to expose the awkwardness of illness and discover a self with new parameters both inner and outer. This ability altered her sense of awareness and relationship with her surroundings; as she relays, "I feel me touching, I feel me grasping, I control the distance between me and objects" (Horn in "Rebecca Horn, Finger Gloves, 1972" 2004).

The work also reveals the debilitating nature of disease and physical impairment when the ability to care for one's physical being is taken over by a complete stranger, the nurse. Often, the ability to communicate fundamental basic human needs can be impaired and there is absolute reliance on the nurse.

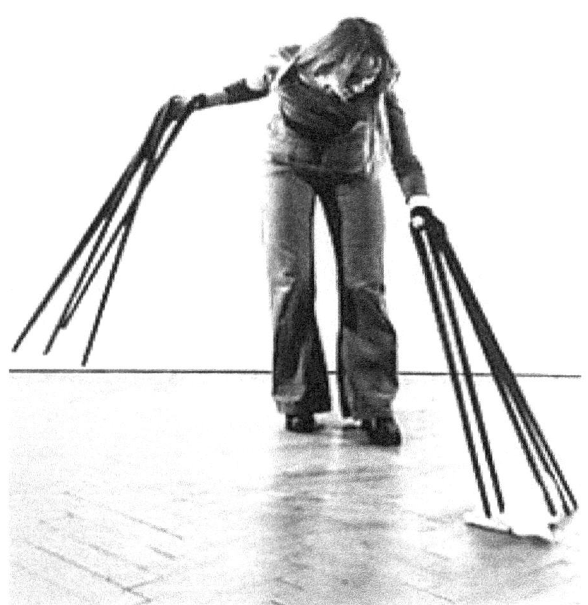

Figure 12 Rebecca Horn *Finger Gloves*

Through this work, Horn also affirms that touch is a conduit for intimacy. Touch has power and mystery and is a complex sensory system, the influence of which is hard to isolate or eliminate. Suzanne M. Peloquin (1989, 18) cites that many writers affirm the communicative value of touch. Edward T. Hall calls touch the 'silent language' (Hall 1973). Jacob Lomranz characterises touch as the initial form of human communication Lomranz quoted in Peloquin 1989). Touch is not only basic to our species, but there is also a biological need for touch that persists throughout a lifetime. In the absence of touching and being touched, people of all ages can sicken and grow touch-starved (Peloquin 1989, 18). Touch is an important component in the interpersonal dialogue between nurse and patient. A touch on a patient's shoulder or the holding of a hand is a potent conduit of energy and is able to articulate support and comfort beyond words. Nursing is a profession where the opportunities to offer emotional support through touch frequently arise. In my experience, holding a patient's hand throughout a frightening procedure can be calming and can alleviate anxiety. Within the complexity of nursing practice, knowing when to touch is ascertained from critical observational powers, intuition, and commonsense. In my experience, some nurses are more comfortable than others in touching a patient. To initiate a human connection can appear to be an insignificant gesture; however, its effects can be life changing and are not to be underestimated (Mitchell 2015).

The value and benefits of touch are evident in the widespread use of the energetic healing modalities of Healing Touch, Therapeutic Touch, and Reiki. These are science-based approaches to healing founded on the premise that the human body has a dynamic energy field that includes not only the physical body but also incorporates mind and emotions and can be accessed by using the hands. While the science-based data around these healing practices have been disputed by skeptics, they have also been positively affirmed by some scientists, among them ex–NASA physicist Dr. Barbara Ann Brennan (Brennan 1990). These healing practices continue to be used in hospitals and health facilities, with positive effects such as reduced stress and enhanced wound healing.

As mentioned above, the deprivation of touch in nursing has increased over the last decade due to time constraints, the wearing of protective gloves and clothing, and, arguably, the use of machines. The gloves form a physical barrier to human touch and interconnection. Since the discovery of HIV in the 1980s, there has been an increasing hypersensitivity to the transference of infection. This gross exaggeration and fear has pervaded even the simplest act of holding a patient's hand, since many healthcare facilities require that gloves are worn in all dealings of patient care.

Richard Prince

Prince's nurse paintings are appropriated from the covers of pulp fiction novels of the 1950s and '60s, which were known for their salacious designs and lurid colours. Prince has taken a skilled work of representational art and, through his individual process, given a new meaning to the work (figure 13). These works would be interpreted differently by nurses than those who are not familiar with the complexities of the profession. The aspect that is most striking in this series of paintings is the immediate recognition of the nurse by her archaic stereotypical uniform, which is an instant signifier of a particular role and conveys an historical narrative of a caring profession.

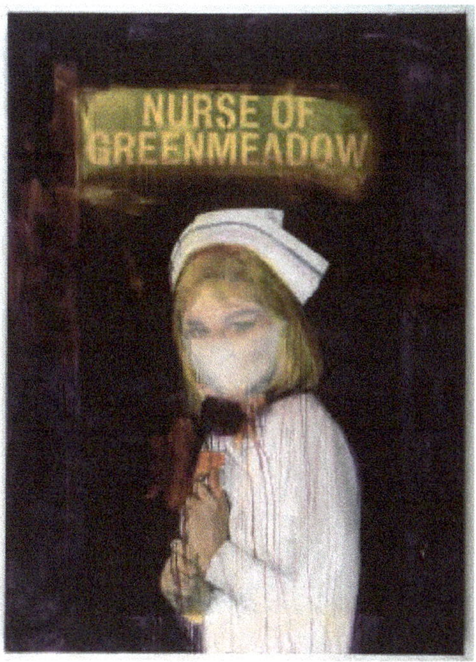

Figure 13 Richard Prince *Nurse of Greenmeadow*

However, there is no portrayal of caring in these images, as the surrounding colours and use of paint create a sense of dread, foreboding, danger, and ambiguity. Red paint drips from eyes, mouth, and groin area, and the resultant images overemphasise the blood and humanity that are integral to nursing work. This could also be interpreted as the negative and painful associations that are affiliated with the image of the nurse yet are not the reality of the everyday. Prince's images highlight the physical body of the nurse, with connotations to sex, blood, horror, and romance. However, they are devoid of reference to the subtle energies of care that are present in the actuality of nursing.

Prince's nurses are ciphers of the feminine—alluring yet forbidden, on intimate terms with the body and close to the profane. These paintings are mythic and sexualised images, reflections of an angelic nurse yet evil seductress. The allure of the partly covered face with a mask has connotations to exotic dancing and the mysterious—perhaps the mystery of a profession that is poorly understood. The mask is consistent throughout the works, being symbolic of the anonymity and invisibility of the nurse. Moreover, the nurse is partially anonymous, unable to speak for herself. Although Prince probably did not consciously aim to do so, these works highlight some of the issues of contemporary nursing. In contemporary nursing, the masks can represent the gagging and silence of nurses.

The nurse is still a victim of the stereotypical view that society places upon her, oppressed in her starched archaic uniform, unable to speak up to physicians, employers, and the government (Summers 2008). These images do not embody or portray even part of the reality of nursing but rather mythologised fantasies regarding the ambiguity of the profession. Prince's nurse paintings bring nursing into the visual arena, which is positive, yet they are superficial, and do not help the serious plight of nursing. They do not tell the reality of nursing, the work nurses do, or address the global shortage of nursing staff. They do not exemplify a profession that is misunderstood with low societal status and perceived value.

William Kentridge

As previously stated, illness eludes easy visual depiction. In his work, Kentridge has used another active concept to explore this resistant image of illness—that of displacement. In *Drawing from Stereoscope* (figure 14), the male figure is in a perplexing situation and we can read this image as representing the transformations of life that occur in the non-visual realm of illness but also symbolic of the visual reality of disease.

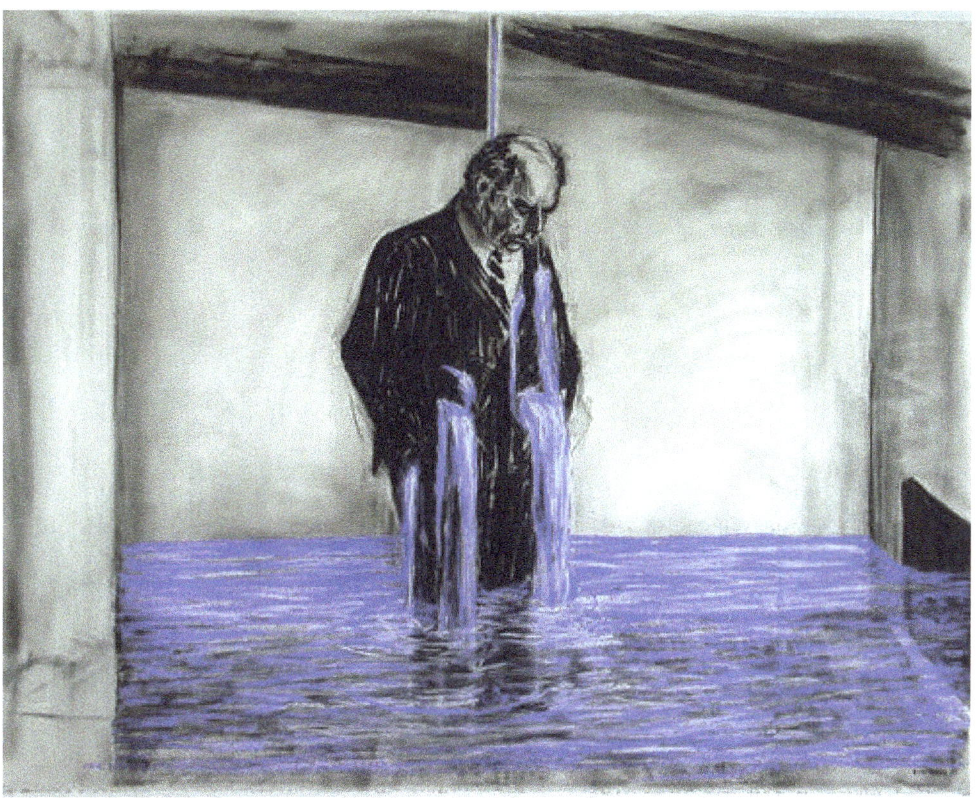

Figure 14 William Kentridge *Drawing from Stereoscope*

Drawing from Stereoscope is a poetic metaphor for the sense of isolation that a patient may feel when presented by the circumstances of their illness and incarceration in hospital. The male figure standing alone in a confined area can represent both the physical confinement in a hospital room and the emotional and mental isolation associated with illness. This image can also symbolise the leaking body. Usually, all bodily fluids are unseen and contained within the largest human organ, the skin. However, when these internal liquids appear on the outside, there is great uneasiness and fear of something untoward looming (Turner 2006). The blue fluid is uncontained and flows from the isolated male figure. He looks down as the waters rise and stands motionless in the face of his fate. This epitomises the fear and anxiety an individual encounters when the internal bodily processes are out of personal control. It evokes the sense of helplessness and immobility that accompanies a period of illness. This is when a dysfunctional body is experienced, and an altered sense of self. There is often an acute awareness of the body, which, prior to illness and pain, is simply lived in and taken for granted. In health, little attention is given to the processes of breathing, digestion, and heart rhythms and there is an unawareness of the complexity of hidden bodily activities.

To visually depict this altered state of illness is impossible, as the tension between the interiority and exteriority of illness and the pain that is felt is purely subjective. In contemporary medicine, the subjective experience of the patient is often lost and abandoned and the body treated as an object to be probed, prodded, scanned, and examined as a dysfunctional machine. The body, objectified and likened to a machine, receives overwhelming attention in contrast to what the patient thinks and feels about their illness, which is often not acknowledged and viewed as superfluous. Often, even after extensive tests, technological intervention, and pharmaceutical support, the patient can still feel ill. As Weil states: "In its every aspect the civilization we live in overwhelms the human body. Mind and body have become strangers to one another. Contact has been lost" (Weil 1939, 38).

The embodied experience of the patient is silenced and unaccounted for, since the human response to illness has little place in our scientifically and economically driven health care system. In contemporary society, the human body is central to economic growth in various biotechnological industries in which disease itself has become a productive factor in the global economy and the body is a code or system of information from which profits can be extracted at the patient's expense (Turner 2006, 223). *Drawing from Stereoscope* also epitomises the isolation and helplessness felt by the nurse in the face of not knowing how to answer or help patients when treatments fail and mistakes and incidents happen. In these times, the nurse and patient face the inevitable in ways to suit individual needs; for example, either with humour or in the presence of silence. However, this image is both a study of dehumanisation and an image of human dignity and resilience in the face of illness and humiliation.

Michael Elmgreen and Ingar Dragset

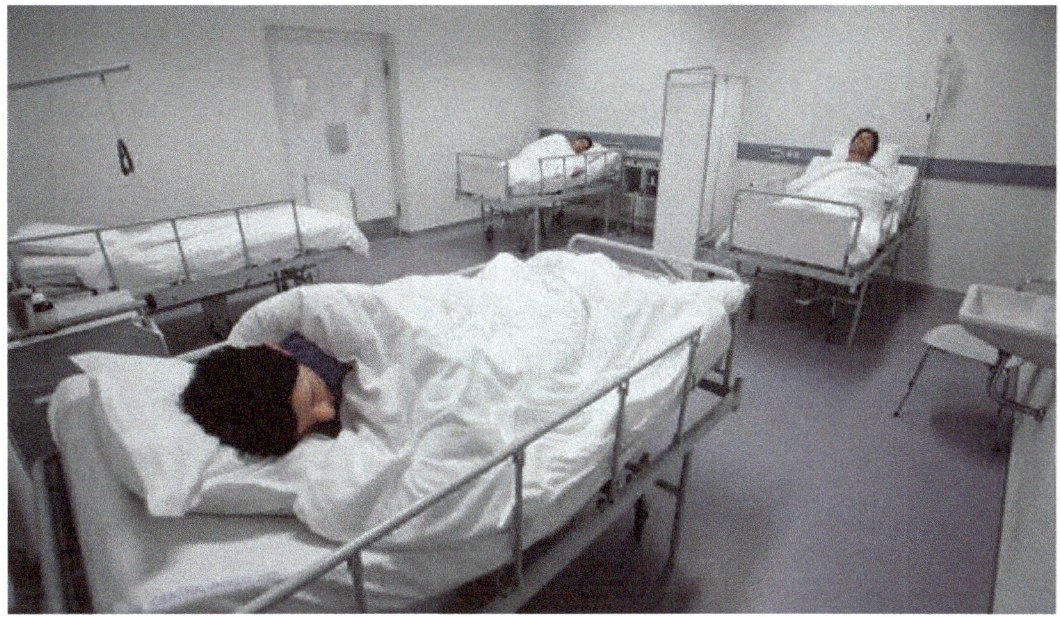

Figure 15 Michael Elmgreen and Ingar Dragset *Please Keep Quiet!*

In *Please Keep Quiet!* (2003, figure 15), Elmgreen and Dragset transform the gallery space into generic hospital cubicles by simply transferring medical objects and dummy patients from a hospital setting into an art space. This installation is reminiscent of a clinical training room for student nurses and would be viewed differently by healthcare professional as it has notions of work place familiarity. However the installation produces visceral feelings of displacement when viewed in an art gallery. The art space is transformed by ready-mades: the objects themselves have not been changed, but are re-contextualised in the art gallery, the power inherent in the objects and their haunting values are evident by the reaction of the visitors.

Visitors from the general public are surprised to see a hospital setting in an art gallery, and approach the installation with caution and confusion as if they are entering a real life hospital setting. The work directs the behaviour of the visitors to the installation as they enter with a sense of unease. In this way, the work is highly confrontational, with inferences to death and dying.

The title *Please Keep Quiet!* suggests an involuntary reverence as silence is required of the general public in both spaces. The work highlights that both spaces share certain similarities of design and minimal aesthetics, being white, clean and somewhat artificial. However they function with opposing differences. The art gallery is a static timeless space set aside to draw attention to artwork that is brought in for reflection, where art is free to take on its own meaning (O'Doherty 2000). In contrast, patients in the hospital setting are trapped in the concrete reality of time and the drama of the hospital space is in a constant state of flux, being a reminder of the impermanence and changing nature of life. *Please Keep Quiet!* draws attention to this dynamic.

CHAPTER 6: STUDIO RESEARCH

My studio practice is directly informed by my nursing experience, and being an artist influences my practice as a caring nurse. Both areas of my life are nourished and supported by each other. The desire to express the elusive qualities of the nursing experience has been the driving force to the expansion and organic growth of my studio practice. This desire is borne out of my concern for the insidious depreciation of caring and empathy that I have observed in the workplace. As a result, my studio research has evolved from mere representations of the nurse and her work through conventional art practices (figure 16) to exploring the ephemeral and actuality of nursing through photography and installation. As part of an ongoing process, my studio research has led me from one development to another in a broad investigation of the interrelationship between fine art and nursing.

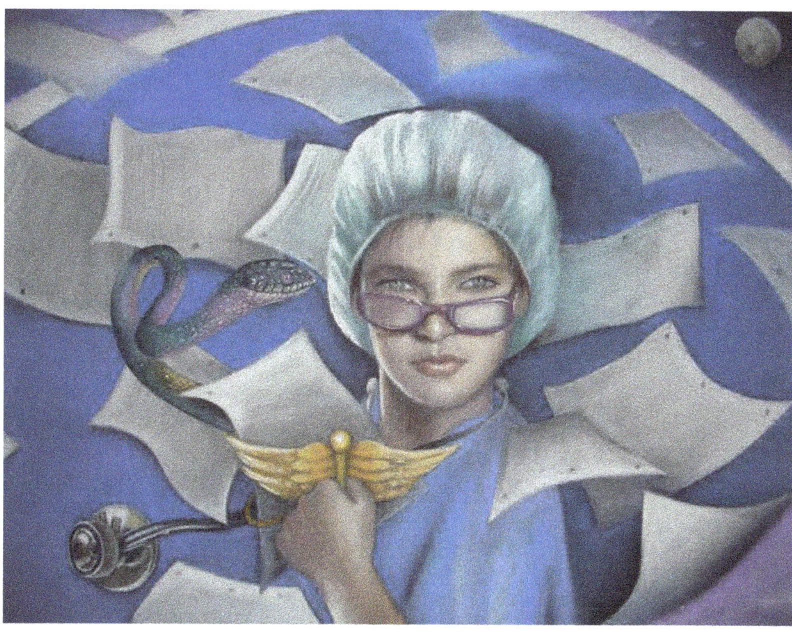

Figure 16 Hazel Cope *Enough Is Enough*

Early in my candidature, I endeavoured to maintain an authentic approach by combining the material processes of the clinical environment and the studio. Therefore, potassium permanganate (an antiseptic) features as a medium for painting in some of my work (figures 17, 18 and 19). This antiseptic is similar in material quality to watercolour, as it is fluid and unpredictable, being brilliant dioxazine purple in solution and sepia when dry, which is also in keeping with the subject matter. Some of my work in this medium is of an historical nature, and hands are a predominant feature.

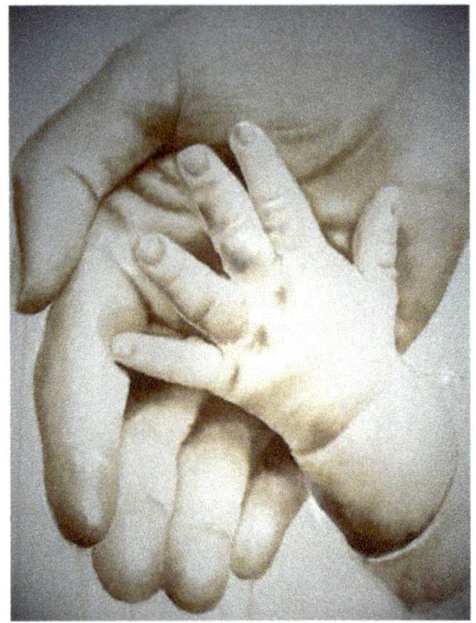

Figure 17 Hazel Cope *Hand Study*

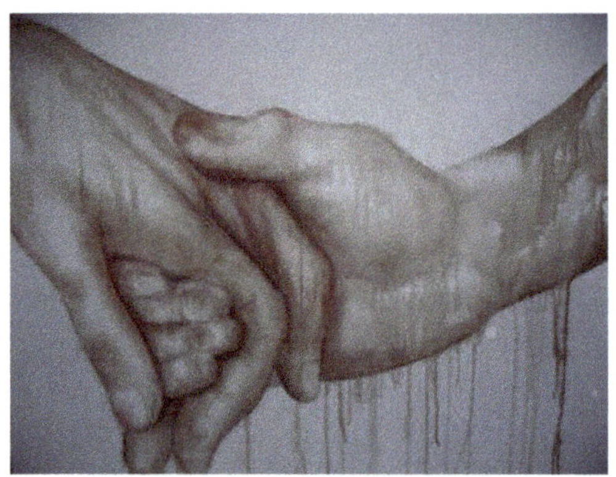

Figure 18 Hazel Cope *Soft Conduit*

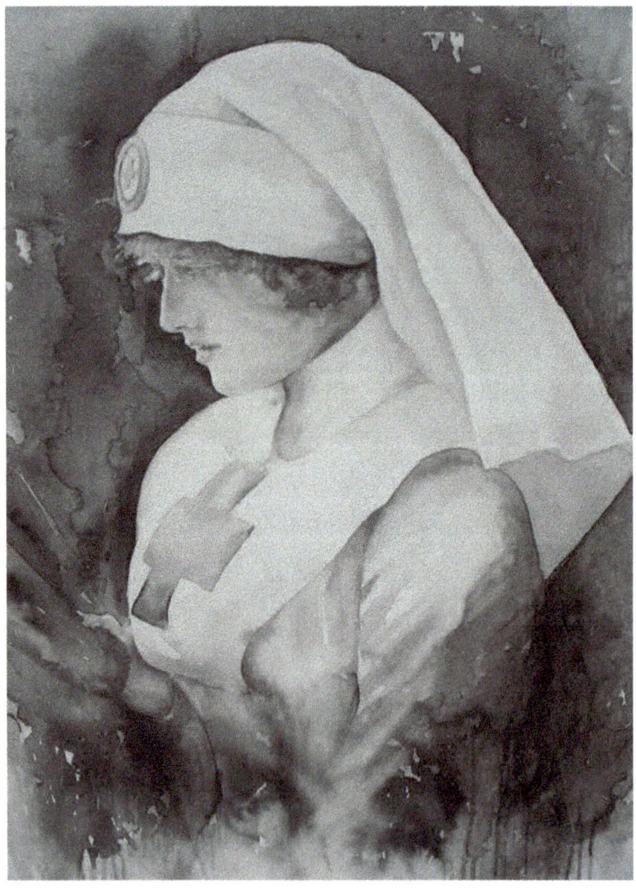

Figure 19 Hazel Cope *Florence Pringle*

I also used charcoal in some of my earlier drawings (figure 20) because of its highly expressive quality. When using charcoal, I need to touch and blend the medium with my fingers; therefore, the work demands a high degree of tactility, which is in keeping with the subject matter.

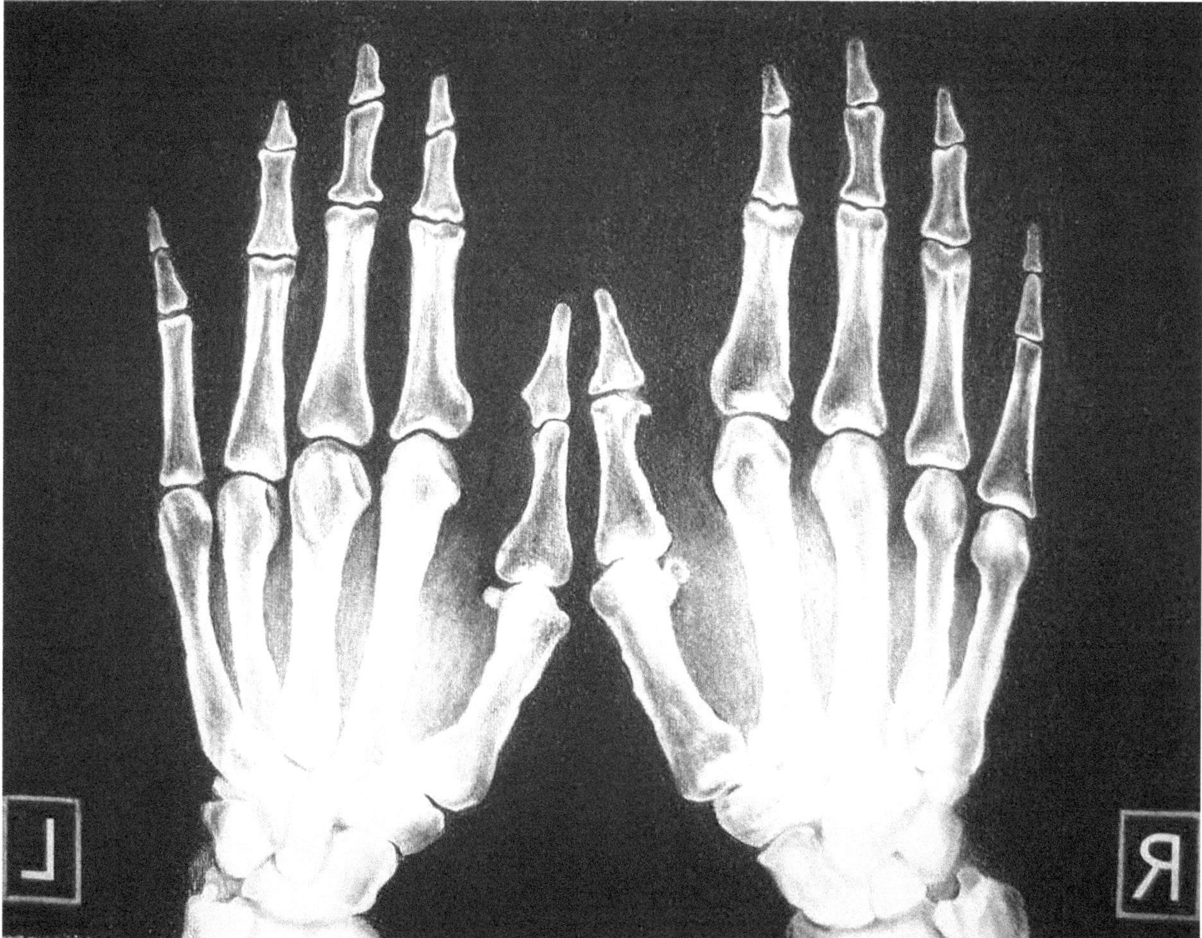

Figure 20 Hazel Cope *X-ray*

In the early works generated by this research, I was concerned with framing the images in relation to the active viewpoints of both patient and those in the medical professional and the use of such optical positioning to explore the power relations at work within such relationships. The pastel drawings accentuated my interest in these unusual viewpoints that nurses have as they make their way around a patient's body to complete various tasks. These drawn works attempt to explore the shifting viewpoints and perverse intimacies of vision at play within the dynamic space of the nurse's physical encounter with the patient's body.

I Should Really Wear Gloves But I Can't Feel Your Veins (figure 21) was one of five drawings I produced in 2009. In this representational work, the nurse's visual field is so focused on the task at hand that the patient becomes a 'vein' that is being palpated. There is visual distortion with intense concentration and observation of the site to make sure the vein is pierced with absolute accuracy. In reality, the nurse scans and occasionally glances at the patient for demeanour, colour of skin, and signs for vaso-vagal attack. In contrast, the patient's gaze will be in the opposite direction from his arm. The pastel medium requires a sensitive application to produce this degree of realism, and the directness and sensitivity of the touch depicted in the pastel image is the very same that is used to create it.

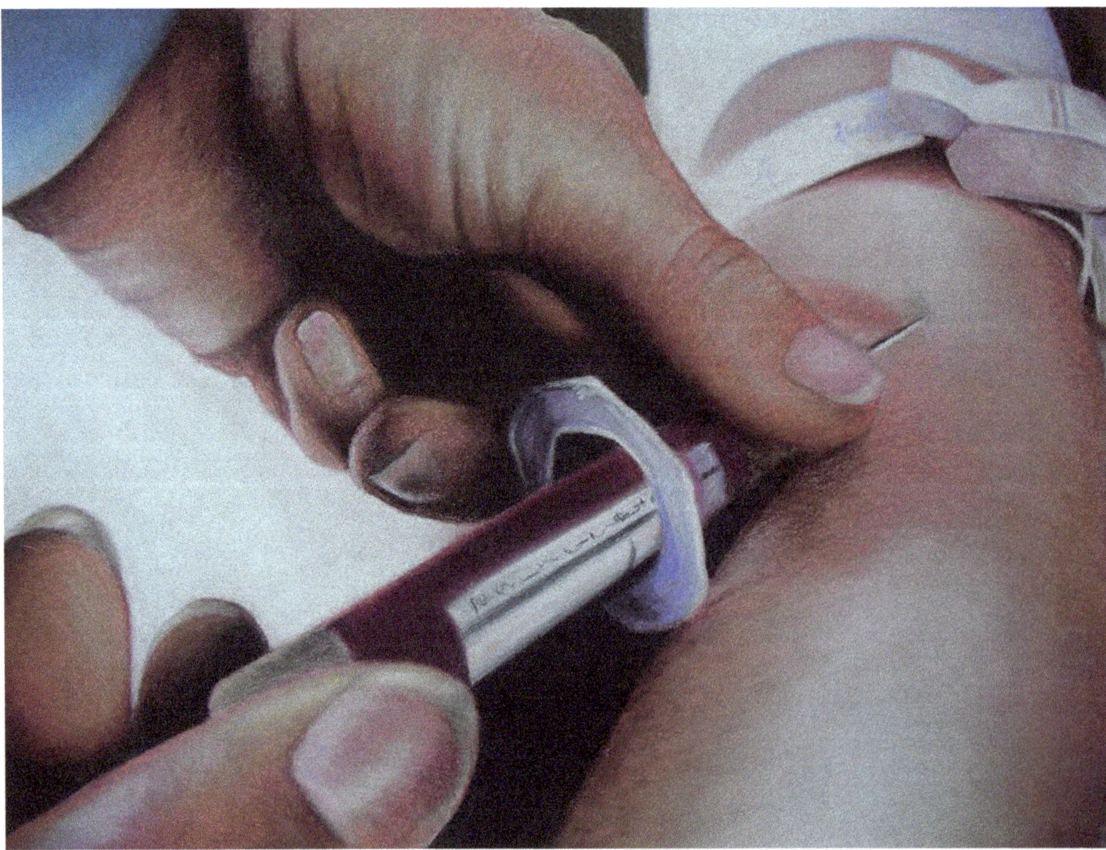

Figure 21 Hazel Cope *I Should Really Wear Gloves But I Can't Feel Your Veins*

In mixed media collaged works produced in 2009, I incorporated medical sundries such as needles, catgut, silk, and gauze (figure 22). These items are the commonplace and everyday items of the medical environment, which are often overlooked and taken for granted by the professionals who use them as part of their everyday work. By contrast, they are viewed by the general public with an element of fear or disgust, as they bring to mind notions of pain and illness. In these works, I have manipulated needles and gauze with acrylic paint into miniature works that evoke the caring aspect of the nurse–patient relationship. I chose to paint true miniature works (less than 10 x 10cm), symbolic of the value ascribed to basic nursing care. Miniature works also require close attention and intimate engagement, similar to the caring aspect of nursing.

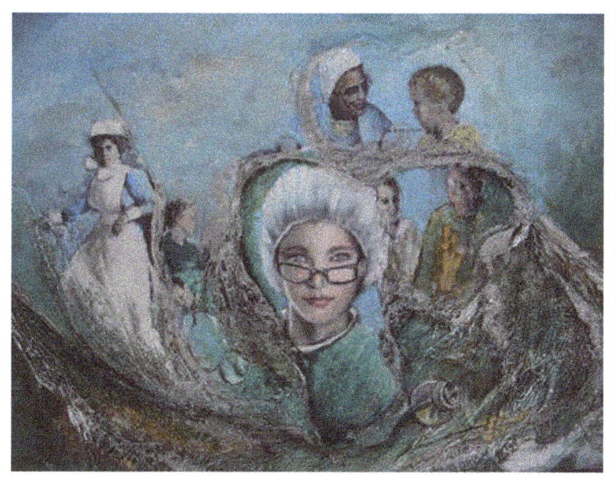
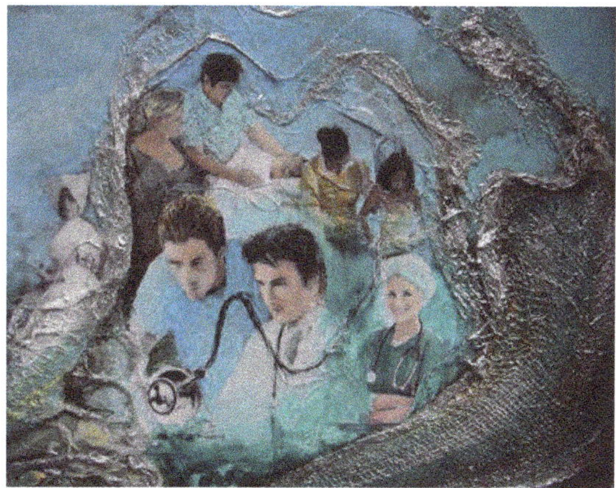
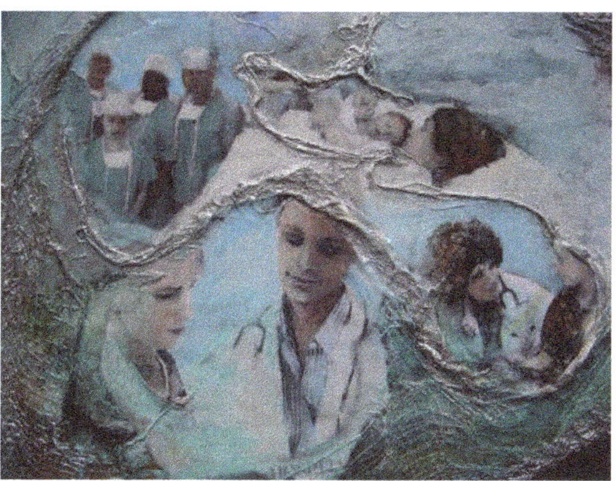

Figure 22 Hazel Cope *Our Nurses*

These works produced at the beginning of my candidacy were well received, and in August 2009 I was invited by the Gold Coast City Art Gallery to have a solo exhibition.

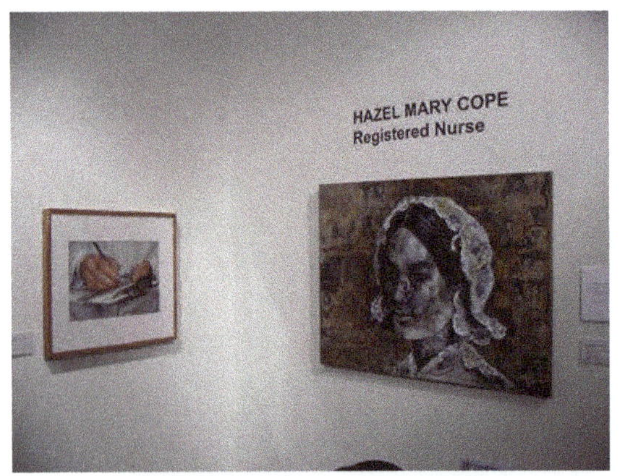

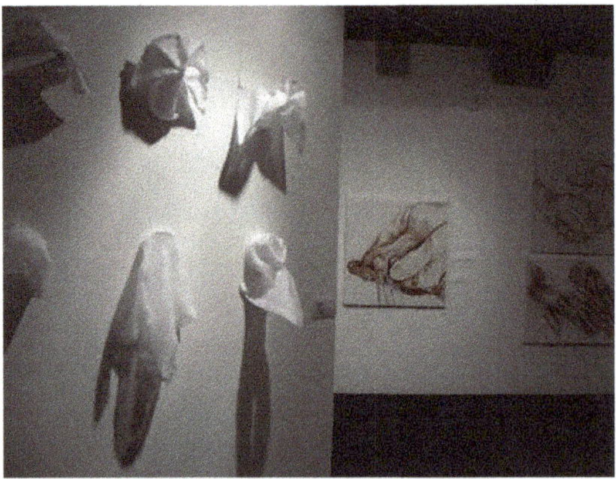

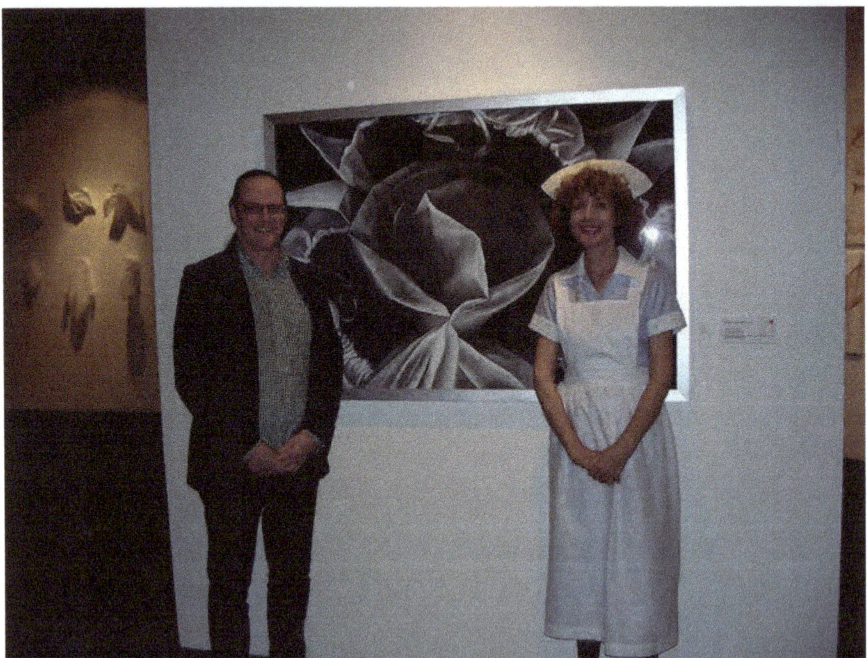

Figure 23 Exhibition of *Hazel Mary Cope: Registered Nurse* at Gold Coast City Art Gallery

The body of work produced for the show, *Hazel Mary Cope: Registered Nurse* (figure 23), explored the concept of caring. In conjunction with my art exhibition, the Gold Coast City Art Gallery held a public seminar, "Art in Hospital Environments". Among the speakers were art and health curators from interstate, including Rebecca Lovitt from Southern Health, Melbourne, and Cathy Hunt from Positive Solutions, Brisbane. Clinicians, artists and project staff from the Gold Coast University Hospital were also in attendance. I dressed in a traditional uniform when giving talks about my work, which contributed an element of performance and humour to the presentations, while initiating open dialogue in the gallery space about the caring aspect of nursing. There was also a display of original nurses' veils from the Royal Brisbane Hospital that were worn in the 1960s, which contributed historical significance to the event.

This exhibition and the publicity surrounding it opened up various opportunities for me, which are outlined in the appendix. Curatorial feedback from the exhibition stimulated debates around the issues of caring and I continued to extend my art practice and create more varied works in this field. In my early exploration of photographic works using light boxes, my first designs were simple, using the historical veils from the Royal Brisbane Hospital (figure 24).

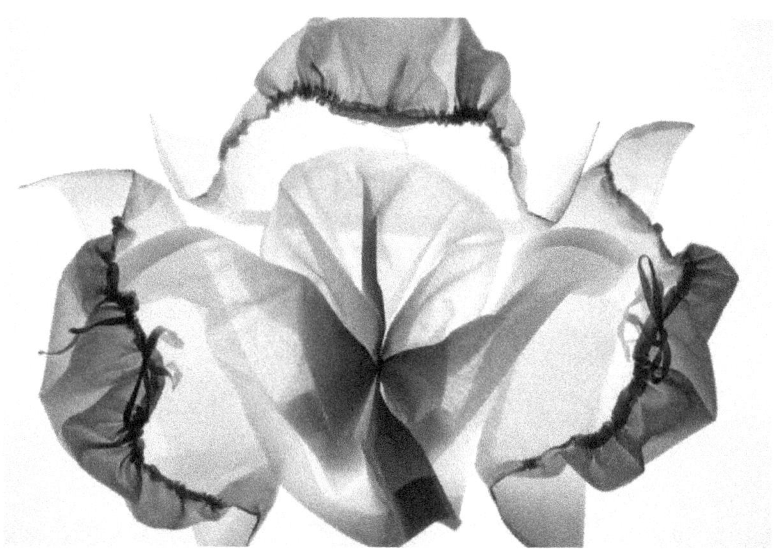

Figure 24 Hazel Cope *Nurses Coif*

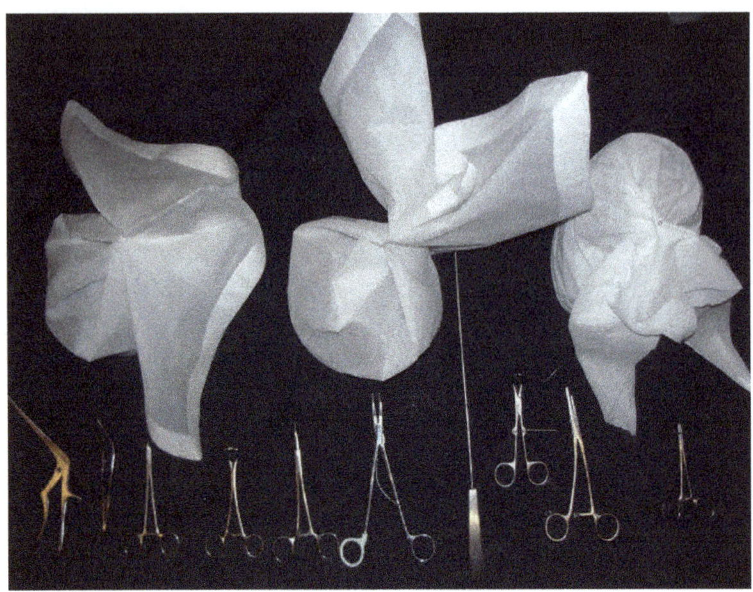

Figure 25 Hazel Cope *Nurses Coif and Surgical Instruments*

In 2009, I obtained a collection of broken surgical instruments and used these to further extend my compositions and explorations both on and off the light box (figure 25). Following my exhibition at the Gold Coast City Art Gallery, I was commissioned along with six other artists to design a public artwork for the new Gold Coast University Hospital in 2010. Our theme was "Beyond the Façade". My personal interpretation was 'beyond the façade of the nurse's uniform, both past and present, lies the actuality of nursing'. This was the impetus to further expand my photographic practice using light boxes and introduce surgical hats and gowns and medical sundries to the works. I again used nurses' veils from the 1960s, as well as starched hats, hospital badges, and belt buckles, combined with disposable masks, hats, shoe covers, theatre towels, and surgeons' gowns, as seen in *Fan 1* and *Butterfly* (figures 26 and 27).

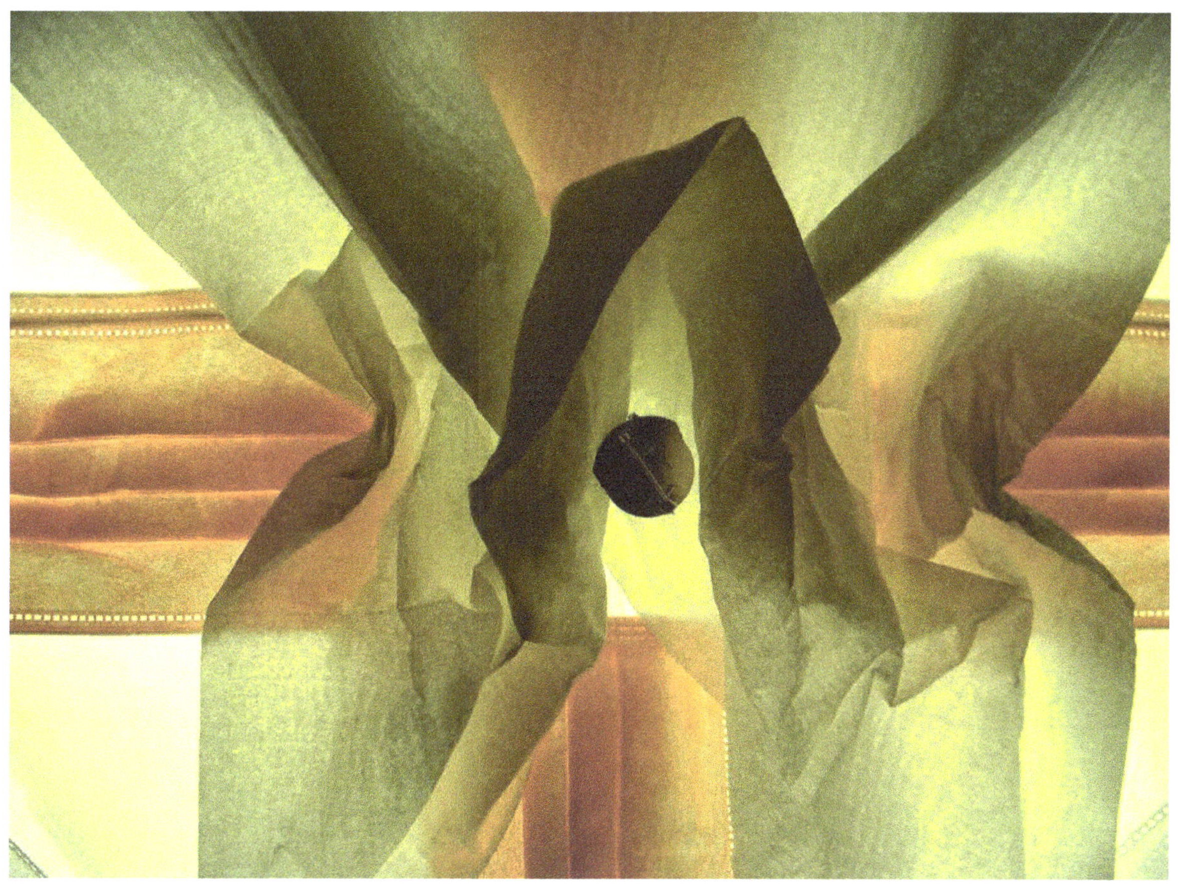

Figure 26 Hazel Cope *Fan 1*

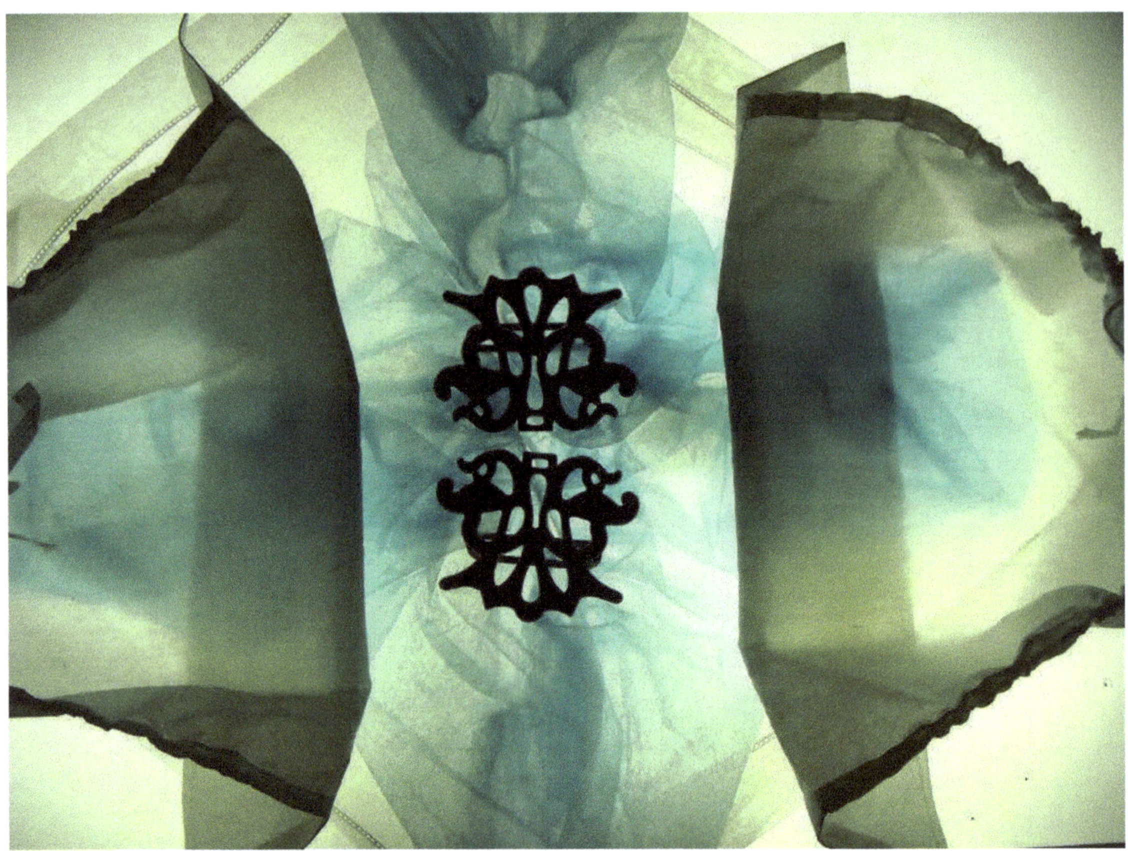

Figure 27 Hazel Cope *Butterfly*

On closer examination, soft organic forms emerge from the photographic work *Butterfly* (figure 27), which is a combination of the starched archaic uniform of the past and the disposable scrubs worn in theatre today. The nurse's apparel becomes something beyond its natural origin (pareidolia). Viewing the nurse's coif from the past maintains an historical link to the great tradition of nursing as the caring profession, the art of nursing. Viewing the disposable items worn today makes reference to nursing as an ever changing and progressive profession. Both styles of nurse's apparel are recognised and acknowledged worldwide and visually define nursing in different historical contexts.

In an extension of my photographic practice, I explored the changing nurse–patient relationship and the objectified body of the patient in tableau form. This involved two photo shoots with nursing colleagues in 2010 and 2011 (figures 28 and 29). The impetus for these photo shoots was twofold. Firstly, in 2010, there was political dialogue and media coverage about hospital waiting lists that was worthy of photographic exploration.

No 42 Waiting (figure 28) was subsequently selected for the Josephine Ulrich Photographic Prize 2010. Secondly, I wanted to explore the artistic possibilities of intertwining the human body and medical detritus in a gallery space.

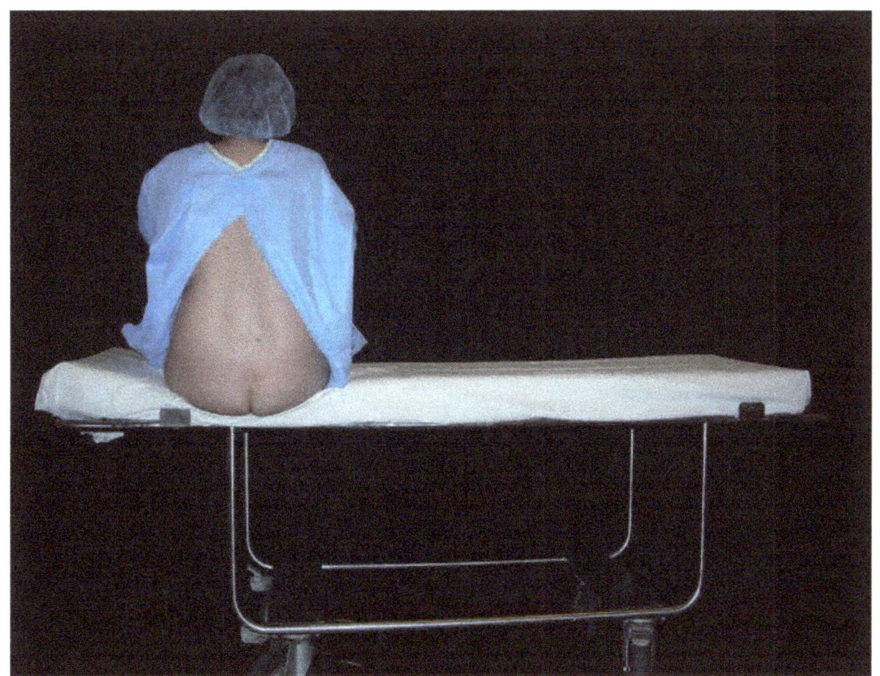

Figure 28 Hazel Cope *No 42 Waiting*

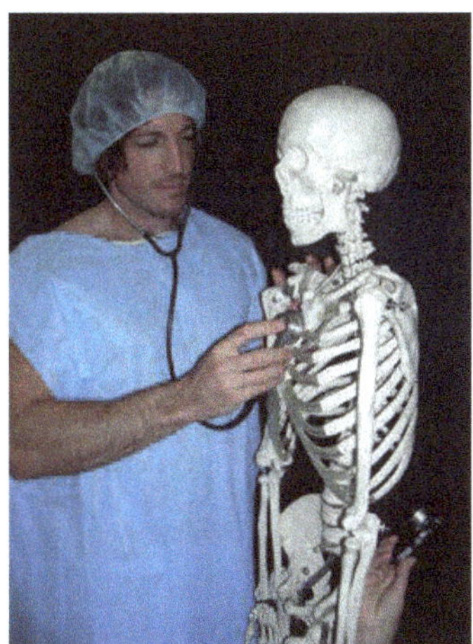

Figure 29 Hazel Cope *Untitled*

In 2012 and 2013, I extended my use of medical materials from incorporating them into collages to making the objects themselves the work, and I acquired discontinued and broken surgical instruments from the Central Surgical Sterile Department of Holy Spirit Northside Private Hospital, Brisbane. My aim was to make various compositional experiments with the objects to solicit their material qualities and to evoke a new relationship between them and their signification. From those experiments emerged two designs that resembled necklaces and a mandala (figures 30, 31, and 32). The three designs were mounted with Sikaflex on wood and secured in box frames for display. These surgical instruments have had a life cycle of their own, and represent the banality of the everyday; however, they also have had a serious purpose. They have been used in graven circumstances and moments of intense trauma in the operating theatre and have contributed to the saving of human lives. Some of the objects have probed and penetrated human bodies, have been covered in blood, bodily fluids, and antiseptic only to be washed and scrubbed and autoclaved once again to reappear on a theatre tray.

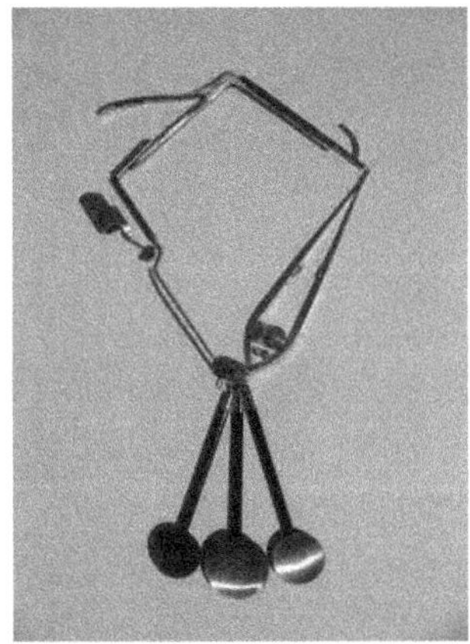

Figure 30 Hazel Cope *Blade Holder*

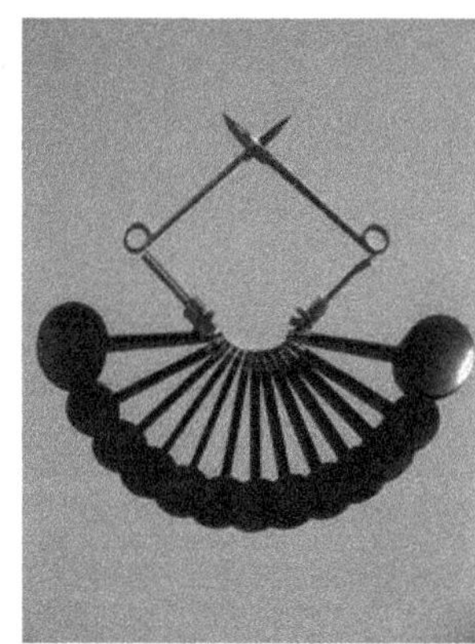

Figure 31 Hazel Cope *Heart Starter*

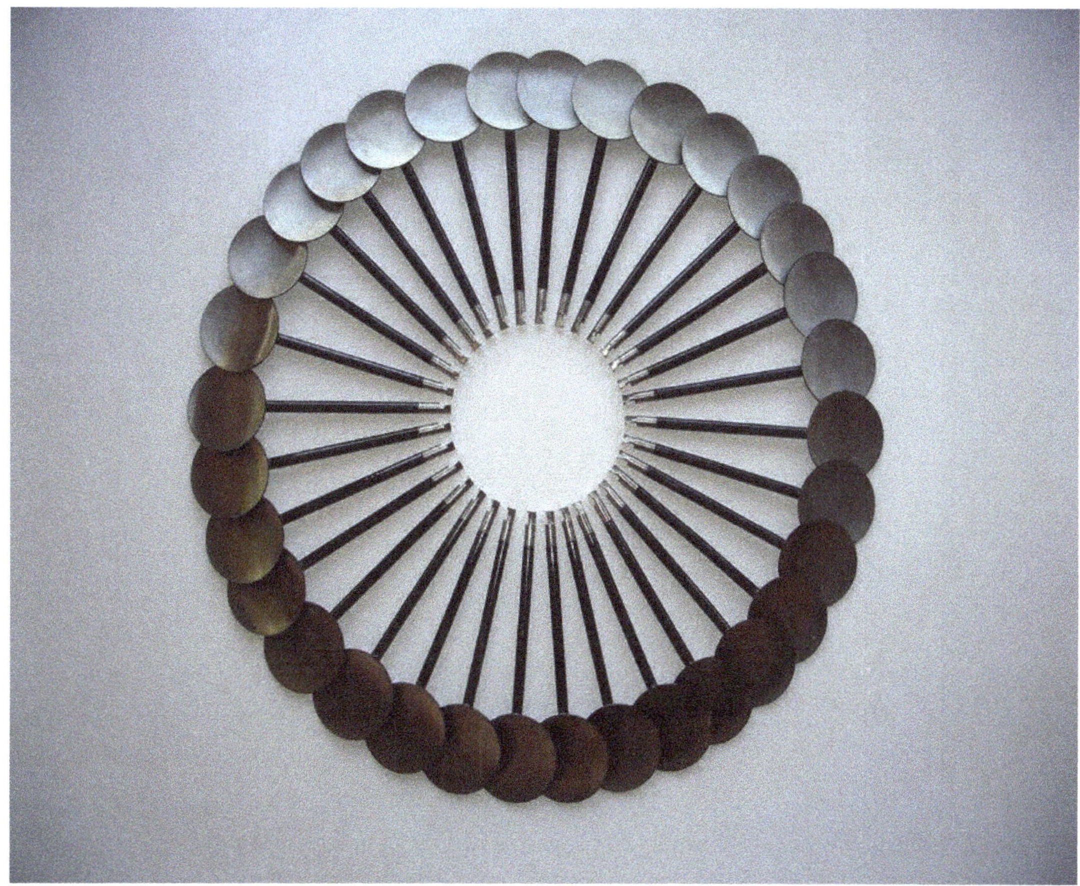

Figure 32 Hazel Cope *Mandala*

Once used in cardiac-related surgery, a single defibrillator paddle has been a conduit for transferring electrical impulses to the heart. However, in *Mandala* (figure 32), thirty-four defibrillator paddles become a mandala, an integrated structure around a uniform centre. The repetition of this single everyday object from the medical environment transforms the paddles into a symbol of sacred geometry and healing.

'Mandala' is a Sanskrit word meaning 'circle'. Widely used in Buddhism, Hinduism, and meditation practices, mandalas signify wholeness, harmony, and the circle of life without beginning or end. The mandala is symbolic of the visible and invisible aspects within the body and the mind. It is used as a visual aid in meditation practices to shift and transform energies and bring about positive change and healing. Similarly, the defibrillator paddles stimulated positive change and healing for patients in their functional usage. The clinical, scientific rationality of these objects is met with a spiritual affective response. Although unintended, the consequence of freeing these objects from their utilitarian driven roles has generated other values of mortality and transference that are often associated with the medical environment in which nurses work. Repeating these objects, there is a shift from the material to the immaterial and a subsequent transformation of the industrial to a reclaimed position of aesthetical power.

The mundane and discarded associated with pain or fear has been reborn into one of beauty and engagement. In particular, *Blade Holder* and *Heart Starter* (figures 30 and 31) have a design element of sophistication and elegance.

Therefore, through my studio research, I have aimed to construct a pathway from the direct graphic depiction and representation of the medical environment to the evocative use of everyday industrial medical objects commonly found and experienced within these environments. I have sought to explore this transformative power latent within the everyday objects of the medical environment through artistic interventions and repetition.

This practice of engaging with medical objects identifies both the unreal or fictive nature of the medical environment as it is presented to patients and explores the potential means of humility and ordinariness within this environment. Furthermore, I aim to return this environment, which is one of artifice and fear, to a more human domain of play, engagement, and being. Many of the materials used in nursing, such as dressings, needles, and masks, are manufactured, received, and stored as industrial objects in a clinical environment and have no apparent or inherent relation or intimate connection to the body. However, when they are used within the space between the nurse and patient, they become significant objects of a transgressive intimacy, determining a new state of this shifting relationship. When a dressing is taken from the clinical room to a patient, it becomes an item of an overtly personal nature, as nurses often have to fit and cut it to size for individual requirements. These dressings, and often devices such as cannulas, directly engage with the patient's body. When these objects and implements are shaped to the needs of the individual patient, they take on a profound, if temporal, evocative relation to the person, despite or even because of their humble and disposable nature.

In making visible the repetition of these objects associated with nursing duties, there is a shift from the material to the immaterial, as well as a subtle exposition and examination of the phenomenon of the total experience between patient and professional nurse. Medical objects such as gauze and surgical masks play a role in bridging this experience between the immateriality of illness and the intense materiality of the body. In April 2014, I began working with gauze squares to make a patient blanket and circular light that I planned to exhibit in my final installation. The patient blanket is made up of over one thousand of these delicate objects that are used in the everyday nursing environment. While they are not given much attention by the professionals who use them, the general public view them as items used to soak up blood and the plethora of 'leaks' from the body after surgery or during an illness. Therefore, they bring to mind an element of unease and perhaps a remembrance of a hospital incarceration.

When examining each piece of gauze in its packet, I noticed that they have a unique character of shape and materiality. Each one is slightly different, which evokes notations of the uniqueness, imperfectness, and fragility of our human life. On the packet, the squares are labelled as 7.5 x 7.5cm, yet very few of them strictly adhere to this. Although made of cotton, the weave is inconsistent, with thick and thin threads in variegated places.

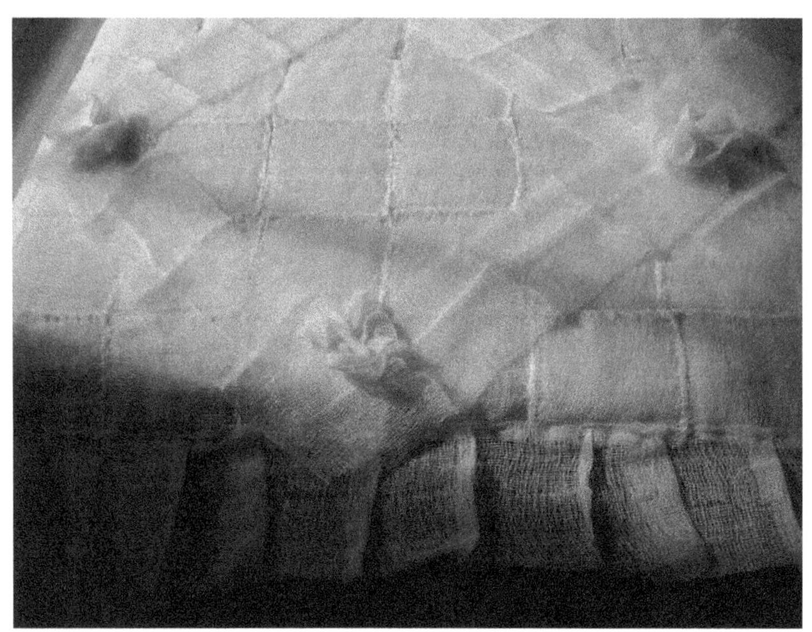

Figure 33 Hazel Cope *Absence and Presence* (detail)

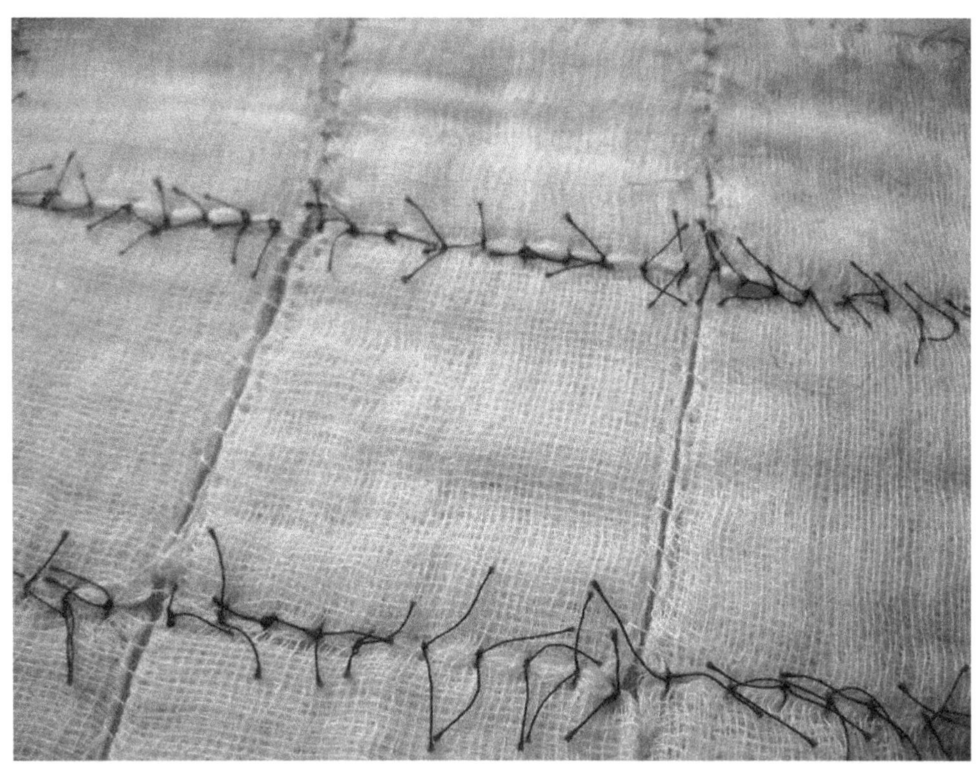

Figure 34 Hazel Mary Cope *Absence and Presence* (detail)

For my work *Absence and Presence* (figures 33-35), I sewed the gauze squares together to create a delicate covering/blanket for the body, using catgut and silk and sewing styles used in doctors' surgeries and operating theatres. Over time, catgut dissolves in bodily tissues, and silk sutures are removed when a wound is healed. Each suture is symbolic of a caring act that contributes to healing. When health is restored, the care is often forgotten, or, like sutures, dissolves into memory. In contrast, the tangible evidence of nursing care is where recordings of patient observations, medication administration, and wound dressing care are strictly documented for legal purposes.

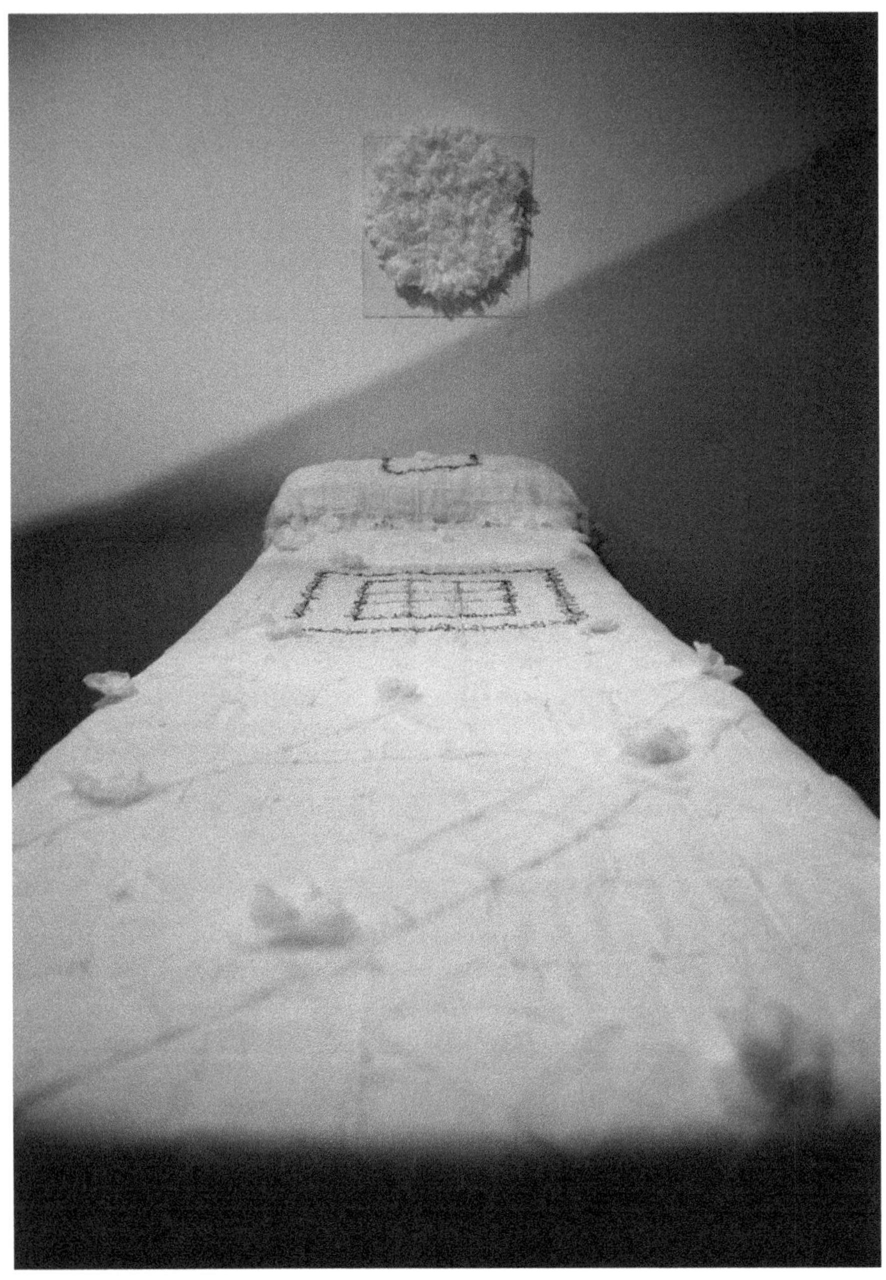

Figure 35 Hazel Mary Cope *Absence and Presence* (detail)

During the tedious sewing of the gauze squares in a regimented fashion, I noted that the delicate cover was akin to the human body in many ways. Each gauze strand is similar to a nerve. In the process of sewing, the needle would occasionally pull the cotton thread, which affected the shape of the blanket. A nurse working on a part of the body—for example, doing a dressing—has to be aware of the patient's objective and subjective experience. This is achieved through an engagement with the patient, which includes dialogue, sensitivity, and empathy, combined with technique, skill, and acute observation. The blanket displayed on an emergency trolley is soft and delicate and synonymous with women's work.

I continued to experiment with the gauze materials and the artistic strategy of repetition. The circular gauze light was made by pushing approximately 250 gauze squares through animal wire with a Spencer Wells artery forceps (figure 36). The gauze squares were secured by stitching and I stabilised the wire with white zip ties attached to a piece of acrylic measuring 120 x 120cm. I controlled the subtle warm light by sewing a yellow disposable gown to the rear (figure 37).

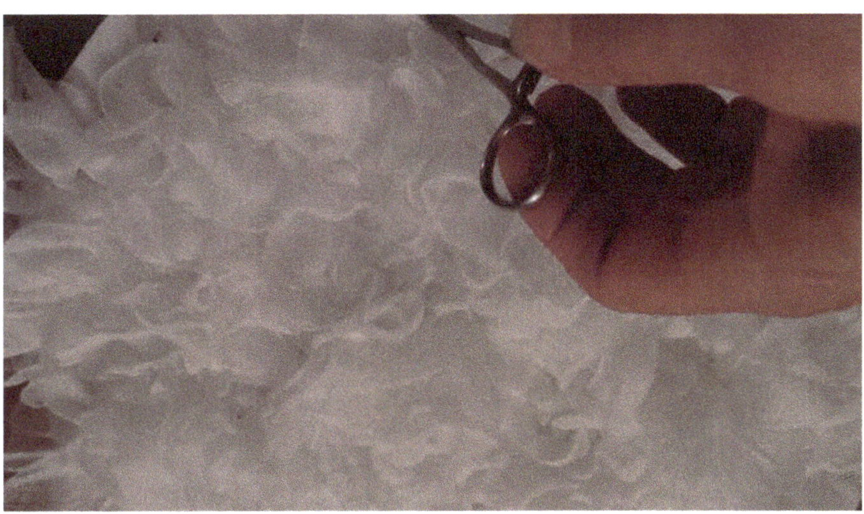

Figure 36 Hazel Cope *Energy 1* (detail)

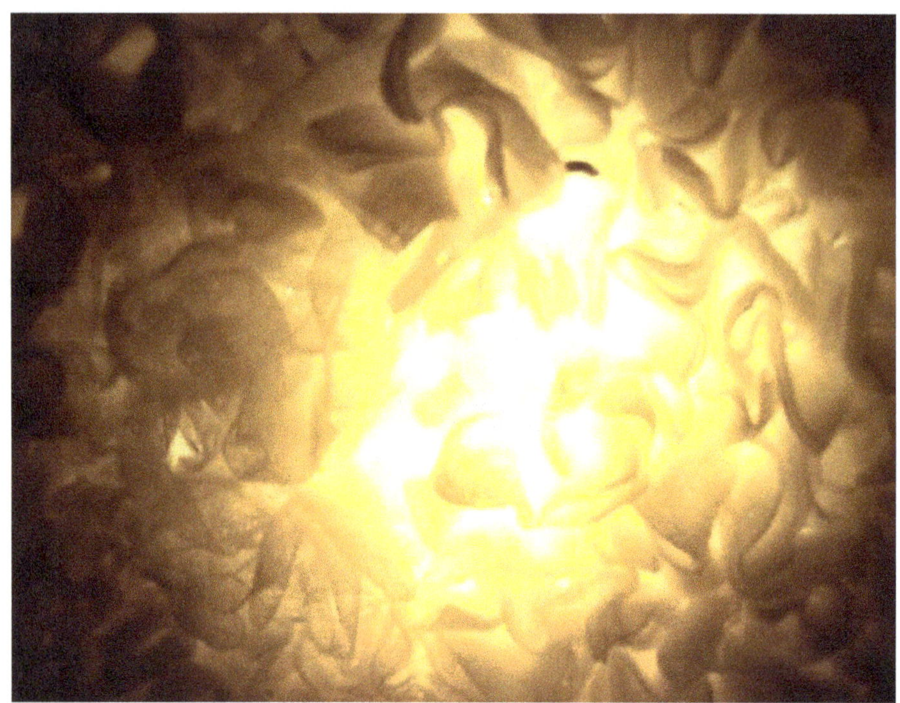

Figure 37 Hazel Cope *Energy 1* (detail)

Further extension of my photographic exploration with the light boxes in 2014 involved incorporating rubber gloves, scalpel blades, and vomit bags into the designs. Furthermore, I felt I could accelerate the process to produce more photographic images by using a combination of photographs from previous photo shoots in a process of layering (figures 38 and 39). I did not use Photoshop but an unconventional manual manipulation. Photocopies, photos, and cut outs were applied with blue tac onto my computer screen. For me, making cut outs with cardboard was less time-consuming than using Photoshop and it worked better than I anticipated, resulting in over four hundred images. The process was also important because it emphasised the notion of touch and working with physical materials. Often, the outcomes were not perfect or precise but have a handmade quality and are each unique.

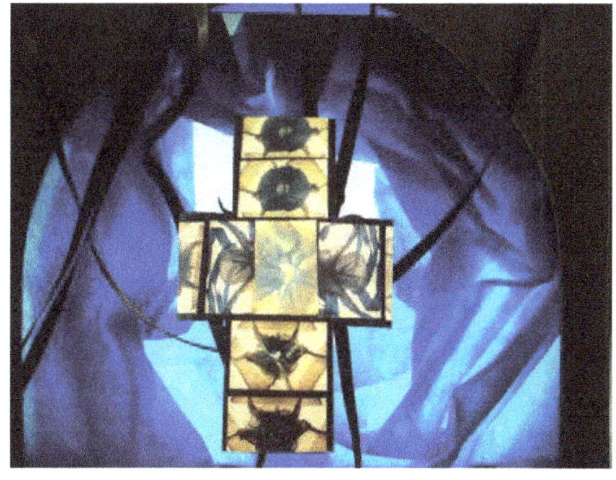 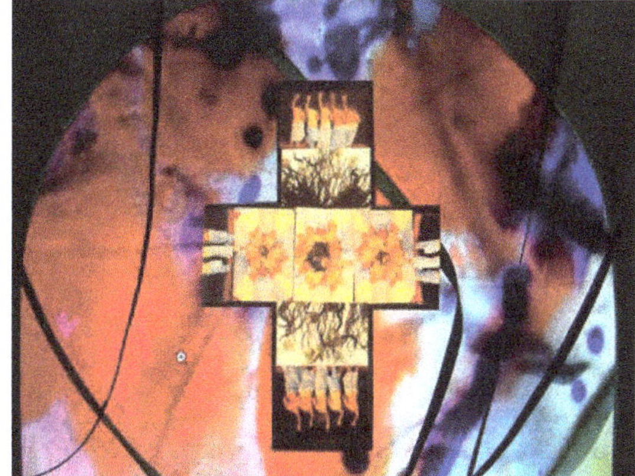

Figure 38 Hazel Cope *Chemotherapy*   **Figure 39** Hazel Cope *Mercurochrome*

The visual results were pleasing because, together, the layered components evoked a sacred quality. Three of these photographs were made into backlit prints (figure 40), and were planned exhibits in my final installation. However, when exhibited in the gallery space on radiology boxes in preparation for the final show, they did not give the effect I desired, as the colours and images overpowered the delicate gauze works and evoked a strong religious Christian connotation. Furthermore, visitors to the gallery, while admiring the content of the banal industrial detritus of the medical environment in the photographs as shown in *Shoe Covers, Vomit Bag* and *Theatre Towels* (figures 41- 43), enquired as to my intention to create a 'religious' space. I felt these works would be appropriate in a different context.

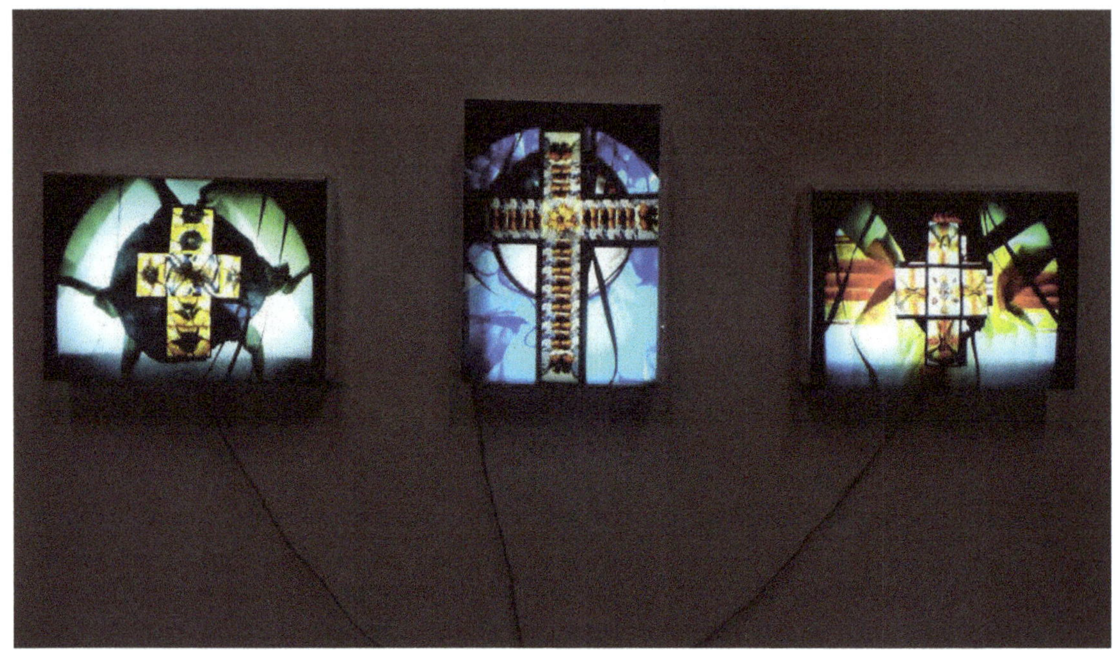

Figure 40 Hazel Cope Backlit prints in situ in gallery

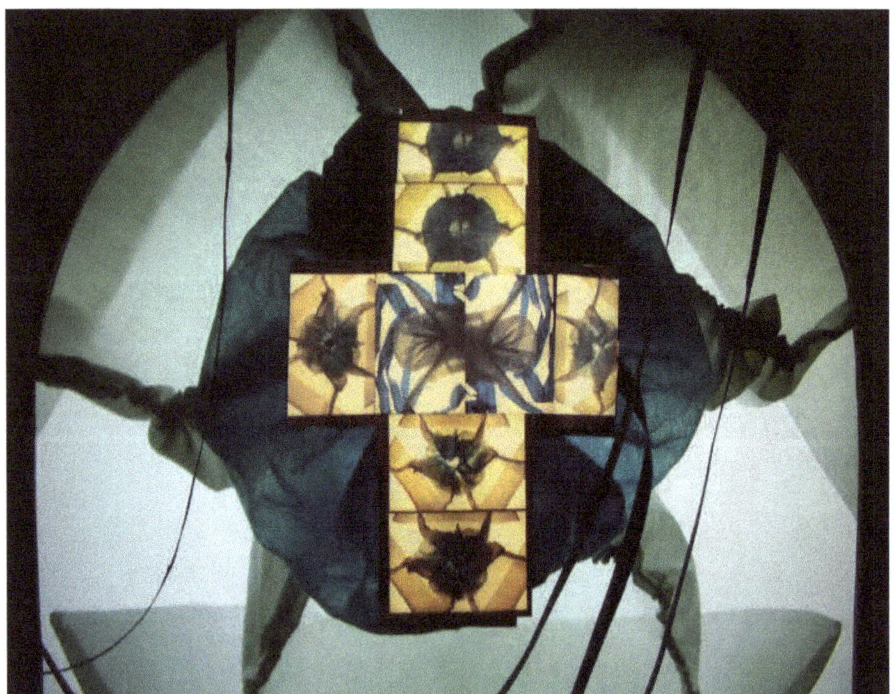

Figure 41 Hazel Cope *Shoe Covers*

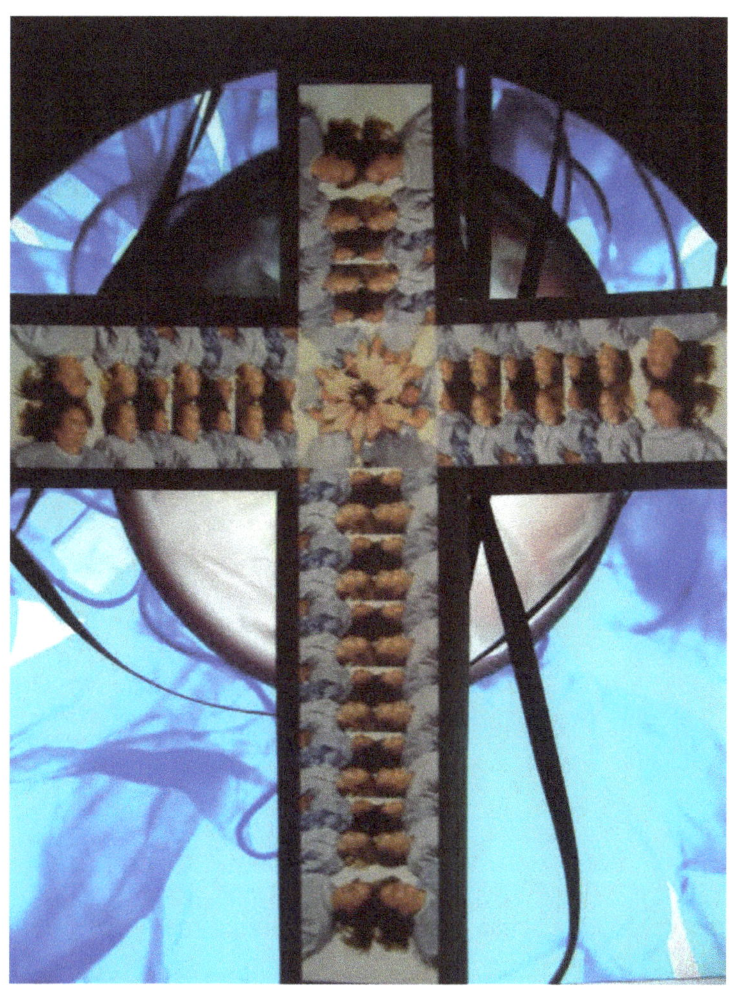

Figure 42 Hazel Cope *Vomit Bag*

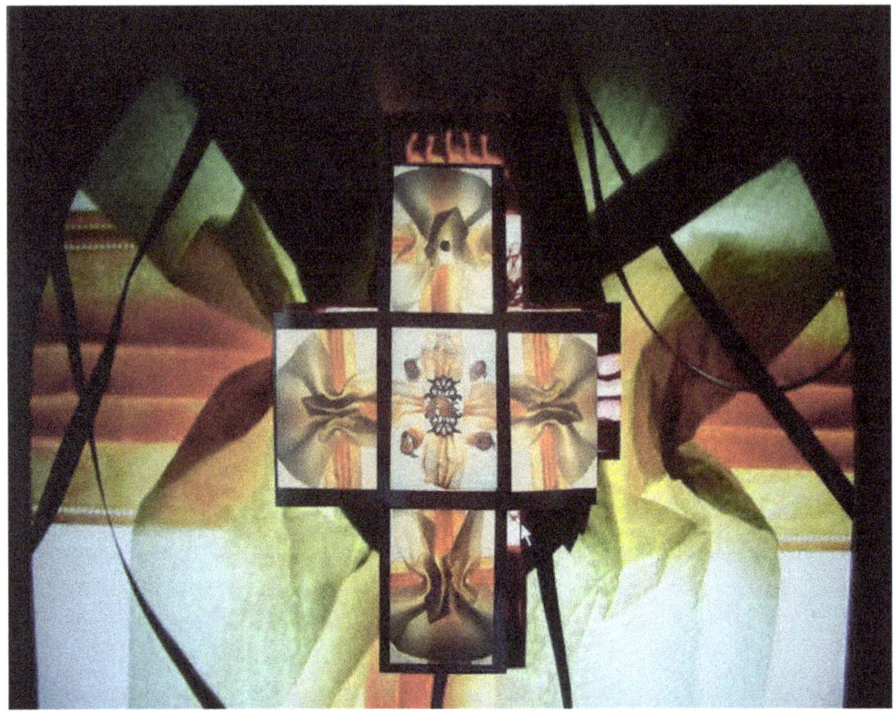

Figure 43 Hazel Cope *Theatre Towels*

However, the effect emoted a sense of the sacred that led me to reflect on the poignant moments in the nursing experience that bring awareness to the sacredness of human life and the mystery of life itself.

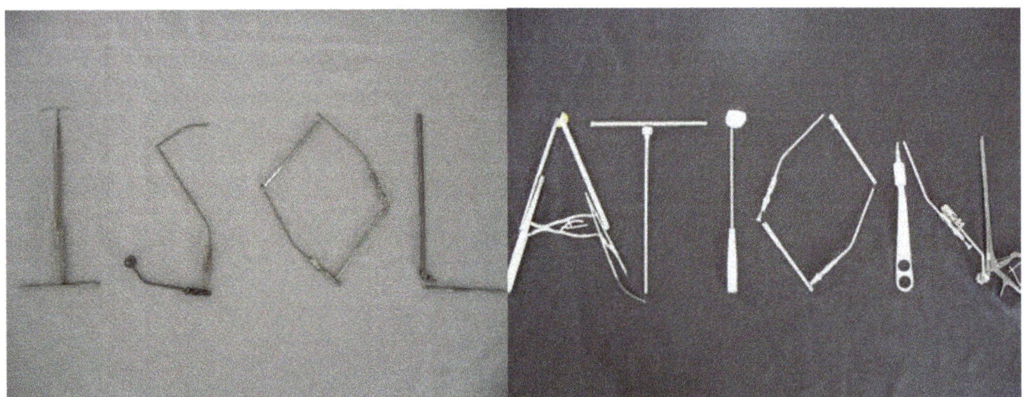

Figure 44 Hazel Cope *Isolation*

In contrast, surgical instruments were photographed on a patient gown without the use of the light box (figure 44). By placing a variety of instruments alongside each other, I formed the word 'isolation'. This word expresses the alienation that can be felt on a personal level during a period of illness; an altered sense of self and a disconnection from a previous lived reality, both physically and mentally. Using the surgical instruments to spell the word enhances its meaning in a provocative and enigmatic way. 'Isolation' also describes the department where highly infectious patients are nursed. The nurse enters the Isolation Unit in Personal Protective Equipment and is an advocate for the vulnerable patient who is experiencing a personal alienation.

In 2015, my final show, *The Mutations of Space*, took five weeks to consolidate. The aim was to control the audience's access to the work and create a physical barrier similar to screens in hospitals. Screens are an integral part of the hospital environment and are subject to the constant rigors of being pulled, manhandled, infected, and splattered with bodily secretions and regular industrial laundering. The screens are a reminder of the fundamental need for patient privacy and respect when nursing interventions are performed. However, the screens I created are permeable, membranous, and transparent, made from bridal viol and petticoat mesh. With a four-metre drop from the ceiling, the screens created a delicate ephemeral presence. I softened the dark ceiling above the patient bed with a piece of organza. The light in the gallery reflected onto the creases in the organza and these shapes of light resembled a heart rhythm on a machine (figure 45).

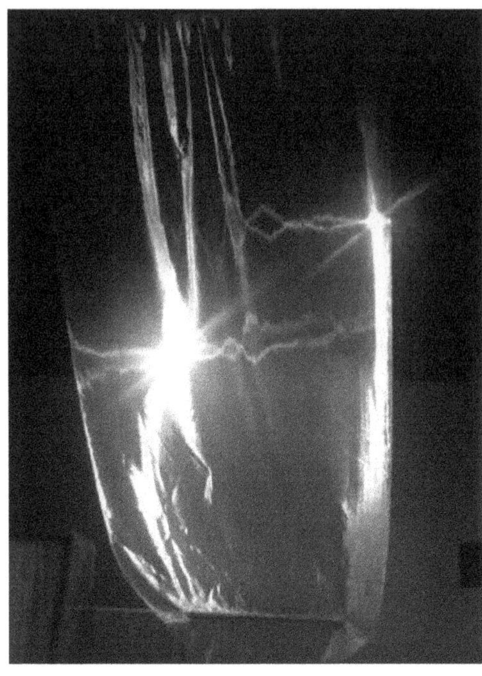

Figure 45 Hazel Cope *Energy 2* (detail installation)

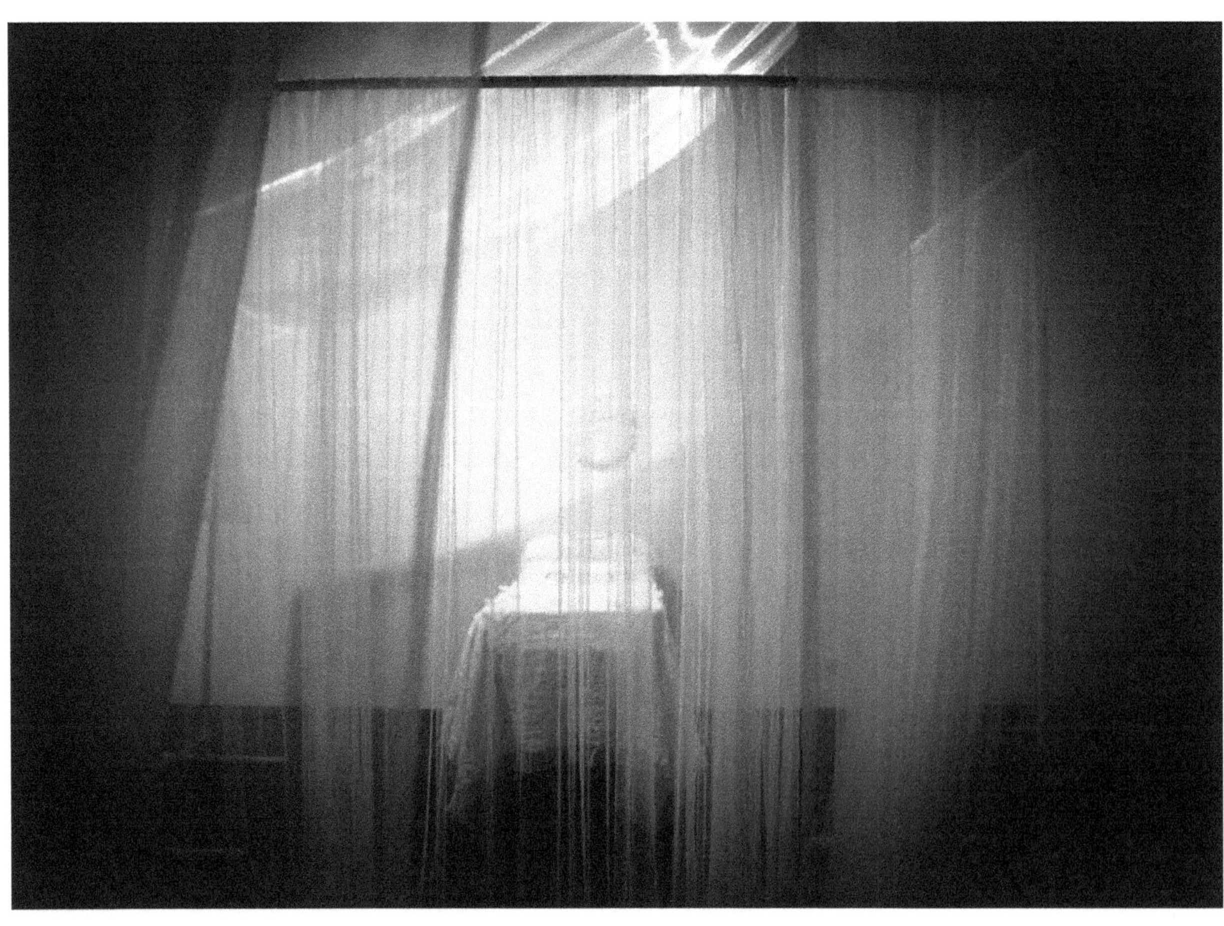

Figure 46 Hazel Cope *Absence and Presence* (detail installation)

I worked intuitively and with no preconceived outcomes. A spaced emerged that is a new conception of a small hospital interior. The central feature in the installation is the textural light (figures 47 and 48), which is symbolic of the nurse's presence, negotiating patient care (symbolised by the bed, figure 46) and her duties (symbolised by the instruments, figure 49).

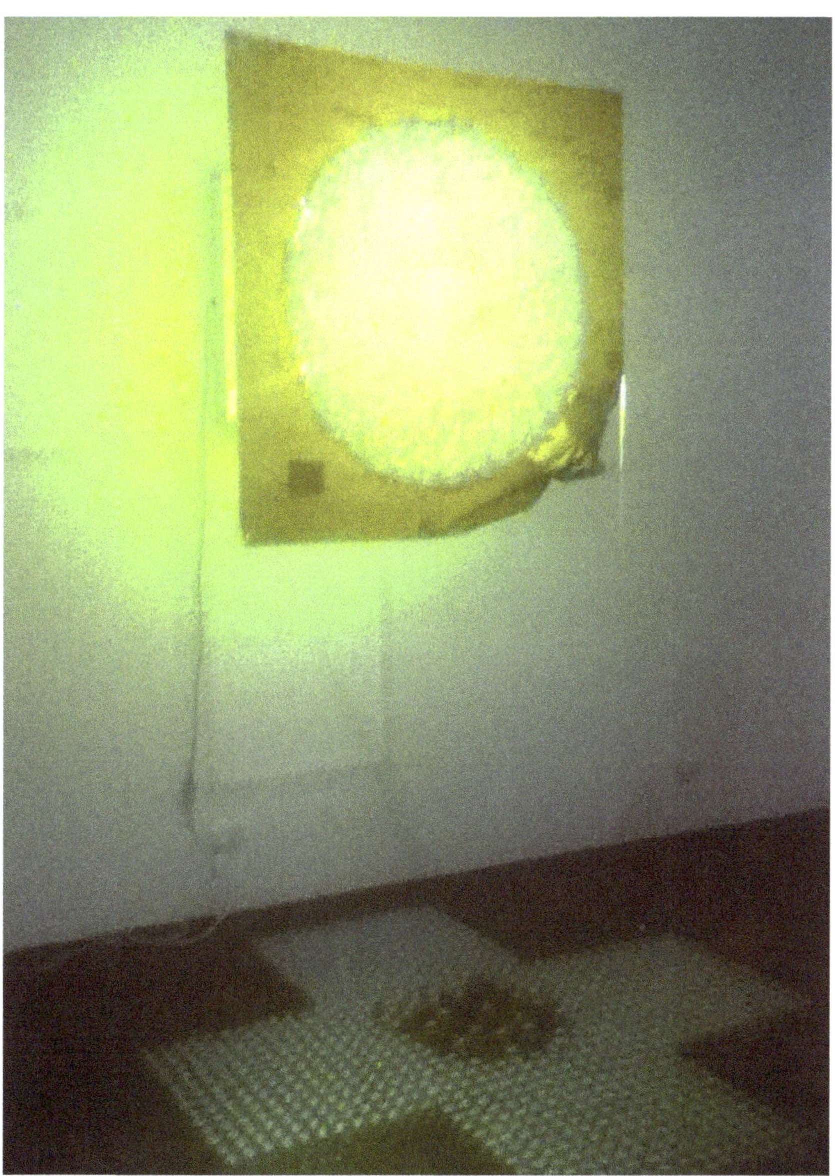

Figure 47 Hazel Cope *Energy1* (detail installation)

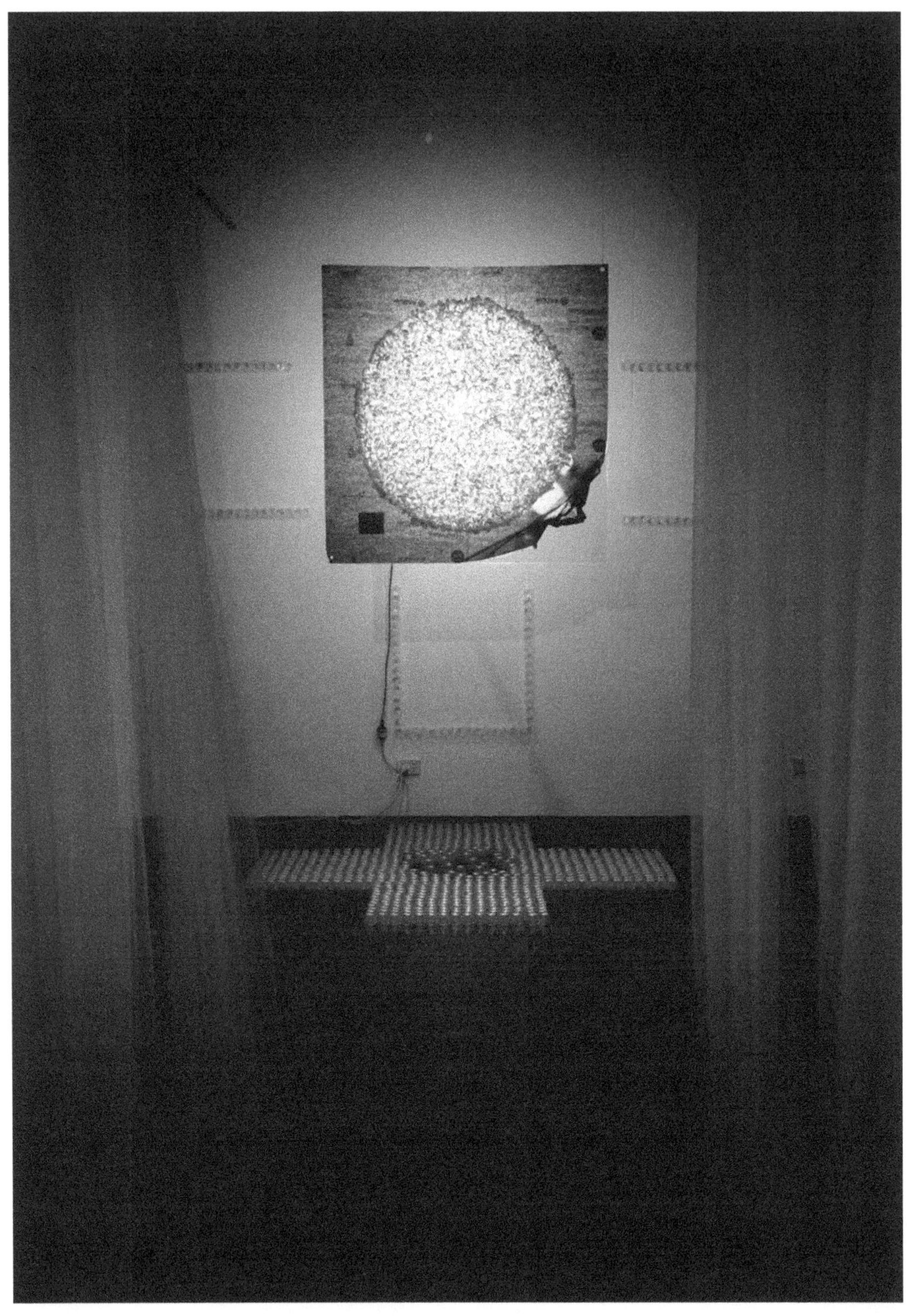

Figure 48 Hazel Cope *Energy 1* (detail installation)

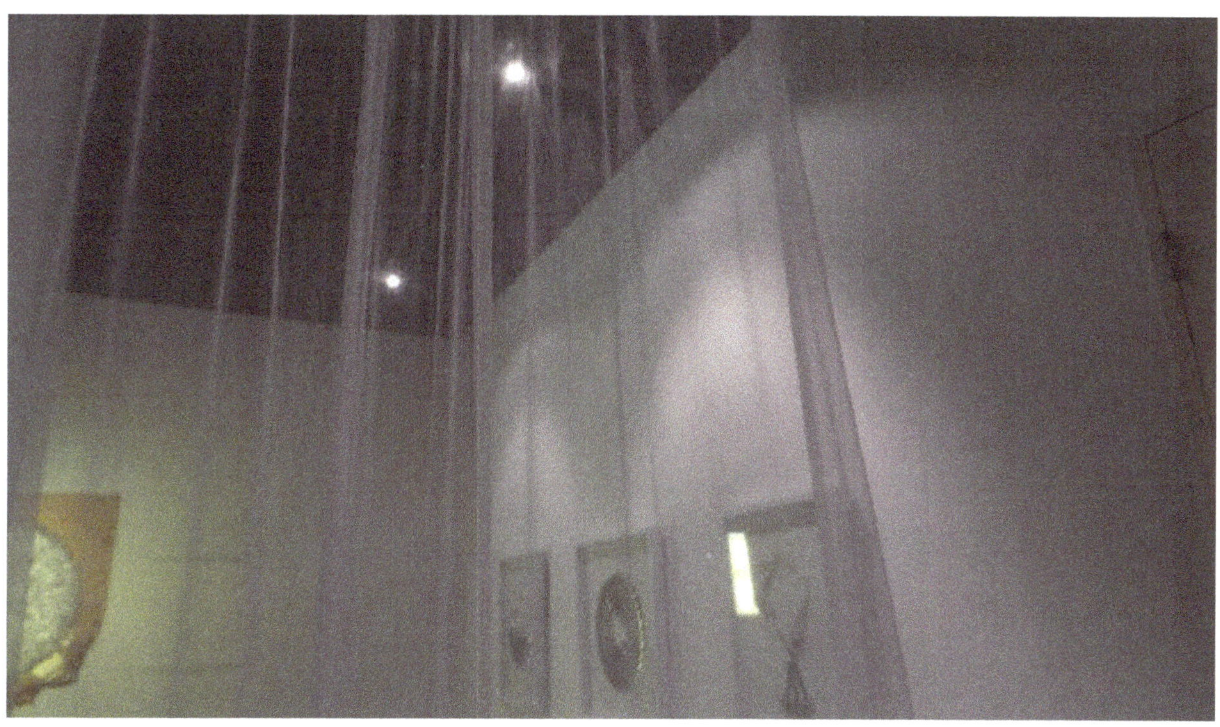

Figure 49 Hazel Cope *Heart Starter, Mandala* and *Blade Holder* (detail installation)

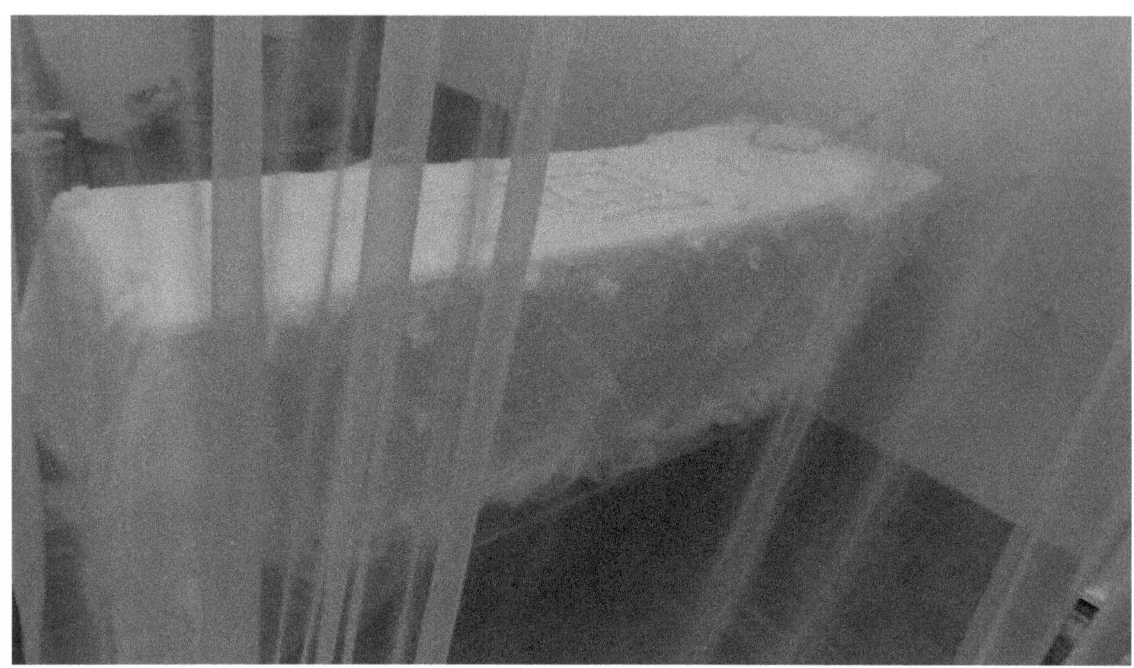

Figure 50 Hazel Cope *Absence and Presence* (detail installation)

The light extends to the shape of a cross on the gallery floor made of over one thousand medicine cups (figure 51). When one passes through the installation and walks among the moving screens, they can detect a subtle antiseptic odour and an audible sound of a heart monitor in sinus rhythm.

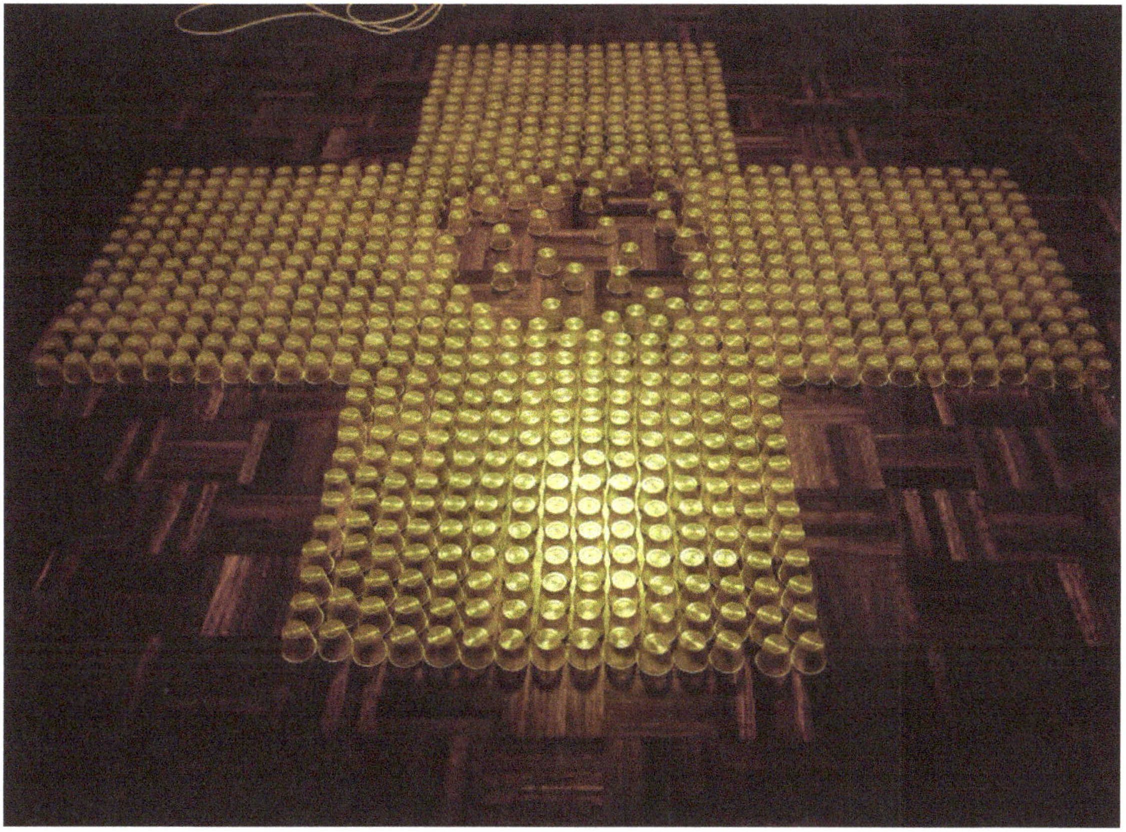

Figure 51 Hazel Cope *Unseen Gold* (detail installation)

The artworks behind the screens are blurred. With the authenticity of the materiality and perceptual activities, an evocative aesthetic is created that draws the viewer into the domain of feeling. Nursing work is performed behind screens, and it is through the vast portal of both historical and changing parameters that nursing work will continue. The subjective idiom in the nursing experience cannot be assessed, analysed, measured, or scanned by medical science or technology; it is in the realm of the unknown and mysterious.

CHAPTER 7: CONCLUSION

This research has brought attention to the authentic experience of caring, which is at the very heart of nursing practice. In my studio research, I have sought to investigate the interpersonal experience between nurse and patient by using objects from the medical environment. These everyday objects used in the medical environment are specialised in their functionality, and they are often viewed by patients with apprehension and embarrassment. In my studio work, I have sought to capture and elevate the evocative presence of these objects to the status of the visible and the poetic through the artistic procedures of repetition and unfamiliar placement. These objects that have been made and designed for a practical purpose are subsequently transformed. This creates a new sensation in the viewer in relation to the objects. My research aims to triumph over and transform the functionality of these industrial medical objects and use beauty as a lever to elevate them into a new space and bring attention to the elusive qualities of the nursing profession.

Illness is an intense and deeply profound human experience felt at an individual level. It pervades not only the physical body but also the mind, emotions, and spirit. Therefore, it is paramount that nurses who engage in caring for those who are ill do so with compassion, empathy, and deep sensitivity. This research aims to bring attention to those nurses who work in proximity to the patient's body. Furthermore, the preservation of human caring is a critical agenda for nursing science to address, as nursing becomes increasingly technological and depersonalised (Watson 1985). Therefore, this research supports the benefits of interdisciplinary collaborations between visual arts and nursing science.

The development of my studio practice over the duration of my candidacy has taken me from mere representation of the nurse and nursing work through conventional art practices of painting and drawing to multi-media installations that explore the spaces and objects of the medical environment. This has opened up new domains for me in which to consider the role and relevance of the presence of the artist in the hospital space, and to further explore and understand the elusive qualities of the nursing experience.

Isabel Stewart aptly sums up the essence of this research:

> Therefore, the real essence of nursing, as of any fine art, lies not in the mechanical details of execution, nor yet in the dexterity of the performer, but in the creative imagination, the sensitive spirit, and the intelligent understanding lying back of these techniques and skills. Without these, nursing may become a highly skilled trade, but it cannot be a profession or a fine art. All the rituals and ceremonials which our modern world devise, and all the elaborate scientific equipment will not save us if the intellectual and spiritual elements in our art are subordinate to the mechanical, and if the means come to be regarded as more important than the ends. (Stewart quoted in Donohue 1985, 468)

Appendix: Research Outputs over the Duration of my Candidacy

Dates	Activity	Title/ Venue	Comments
31 July–6 September 2009	Solo art exhibition	*Hazel Mary Cope: Registered Nurse,* Gold Coast City Art Gallery, Gold Coast, QLD	
December 2009	Regional Arts Development Grant	*Hazel Mary Cope: Registered Nurse.* Catalogue for a solo art exhibition at Logan Regional Art Gallery, Logan, QLD	
December 2009	Publication in *Connections,* Journal of the Royal College of Nursing, Australia	"The Art and Science of Caring" *Connections* 12(2) Front Cover: page 22	
6 February 2010	Photos shoot with nursing colleagues	White Box Gallery, Griffith University, Gold Coast, QLD	
12 February–13 March 2010	Solo art exhibition	*Spotlight on Nurses,* Logan Regional Art Gallery, Logan, QLD	
April 2010	Commission: Design public artwork for the new Gold Coast University Hospital, Gold Coast QLD	Creative Sight 255 Gregory Terrace, Brisbane, QLD	
9 April–23 May 2010	Selection: *No 42. Waiting*	Josephine Ulrick and Win Schubert Photography Award, Gold Coast City Art Gallery, Gold Coast, QLD	
September 2010	Selection: *Inside our Hospice*	Mortimore Art Prize Exhibition, touring Australia	

10 September 2010	Television Interview	Griffith Film School, Griffith University, Brisbane, QLD	
January 2011	Selection: *Celebration of Nursing, Scrub Nurse, Skilled Midwife 1 and 2, Soft Conduit.*	*Nursing the Finest Art: An Illustrated History* by Dr. Patricia Donahue	Largest illustrated book in the world depicting the history of nursing. New edition 2013.
January 2011	Commission: Ten A1 digital photographs. *Nurses Coif 1960s*	Medical Imaging Department, Mater Hospital, Brisbane, QLD	
6 March–12 July 2011	Solo art exhibition	Wesley Hospital, Brisbane, QLD	
17 May–3 June 2011	Selection: *Night Nurse*	Northern Rivers Portrait Prize, Salon Des Refuses, Serpentine Gallery, Lismore, NSW	
9 June 2011	Photo shoot with nursing colleagues	White Box Gallery, Griffith University, Gold Coast, QLD	
November 2011	Selection: *Washing Hands, Nurses Coif 1960s*	Saatchi permanent online Museum Gallery, London, UK	
March 2012	Solo art exhibition	Red Cross Blood Bank, Gold Coast, QLD	
September 2012	Solo art exhibition	St Vincent's Hospital Toowoomba, QLD	St Vincent's Hospital produced a catalogue *Celebration of Care* featuring selected artworks combined with a history of 90 years of care in the Darling Downs Region. Toowoomba, QLD
September 2012	Television article about art exhibition	Toowoomba, QLD	
December 2012		Made Honorary Member of	

		Canadian-based *Art by Nurses* an online art gallery	
March 2013	Purchase of three A1 digital photographs *Fan, Old and New, Masks*	Gold Coast University Hospital Art Collection, Gold Coast, QLD	
September 2013	Solo art exhibition	Holy Spirit Northside Private Hospital, Brisbane, QLD	Catalogue: *The Art of Caring*
3 August 2014	Featured artist book launch	Mark Hunter World Toastmaster 2009, *Voice of the Bonsai* Ross Evans Centre, Gold Coast, QLD	
October 2014–February 2016	Solo art exhibition	St Joseph's Monastery, Oxford Park, Brisbane, QLD	
3 January–16 February 2015	Solo art exhibition *The Mutations of Space* preparation for final art installation Doctor of Visual Arts examination	White Box Gallery, Griffith University, Gold Coast, QLD	

REFERENCES

Australian Bureau of Statistics. 2013. *Doctors and Nurses Australian Social Trends.*
http://www.abs.gov.au/AUSSTATS/abs@.nfs/Lookup/4102.OMain+Features.

Balls, Paula. 2009. "Phenomenology in Nursing Research: Methodology, Interviewing and Transcribing." *Nursing Times* 105(32–33): 30–33.

Benjamin, Walter. 1936. "The Work of Art in the Age of Mechanical Reproduction." Translated by Harry Zohn. *Marxist Internet Archive.*
marxists.org /reference/subject/philosophy/works/ge/benjamin.htm.

Benner, Patricia, Christine Tanner, and Catherine Chesla. 2009. *Expertise in Nursing Practice.* New York: Springer Publishing Company.

Brennan, Barbara Ann. 1990. *Hands of Light: A Guide to Healing through the Human Energy Field.* New York: Bantam Publishing.

Buck-Morss, Susan. 1992. "Aesthetics and Anesthetics: Walter Benjamin's Artwork Essay Reconsidered." *October* 62: 3–41.

Cluff, Leighton E., and Robert Binstock. 2001. *The Lost Art of Caring.* Baltimore: John Hopkins University Press.

Donahue, Patricia. 1985. *Nursing, The Finest Art: An Illustrated History.* St. Louis, MO: Mosby Company.

Dubroff, M. Dee. 2010. "Japanese Robots Become Hospital Staff." *Weird Asia News*, 13 November.
http://www.weirdasianews.com/2010/11/13japanese-robots-hospital-staff/.

Dyer, Jennifer. 2009. "Review of *The Everyday*, ed. Stephen Johnstone." *Invisible Culture: An Electronic Journal for Visual Culture* 13.
https://www.rochester.edu/in_visible_culture/Issue_13_/reviews/dyer.html.

"Everyday." *Wikipedia*, last updated 13 July 2015. http://enwikipedia.org/wiki/Everyday_life.

Formis, Barbara. 2004. "Event and Readymade: Delayed Sabotage." *Communication and Cognition* 37: 247–61.

Foucault, Michel. 1973. *Birth of the Clinic.* London: Routledge.

Gendlin, Eugene. 1959. The Focusing Institute Inc.
http://www.focusing.org/gendlin/docs/gol_2077.html.

Hall, Edward T. 1973. *The Silent Language.* New York: Anchor.

Haynes, Deborah J. 1997. *The Vocation of the Artist.* New York: Cambridge University Press.

Hudson-Jones, Anne. 1988. *Images of Nurses: Perspectives from History, Art, and Literature.* Philadelphia: University of Pennsylvania Press.
Johnstone, Stephen, ed. 2008. *The Everyday.* London: Whitechapel Gallery.

Jung, Carl. 1961. *Memories, Dreams and Reflections.* London: Fontana.

Koh, Germaine. 2005. *Knitwork.* http://www.germainekoh.com/ma/projects_details.cfm?pg=projects&projectID==87.

Kossolapow, Line, Sarah Scoble, and Diane Waller, eds. 2003. *Arts – Therapies – Communication.* Berlin: LIT Verlag.

Krysl, Marilyn. 2012. "Writing the Caring Experience." *Marilyn Krysl* (website). http://www.marilynkrysl.com/krysl/nursing.html.

Kuhse, Helga. 1997. *Caring: Nurses, Women and Ethics.* Oxford: Blackwell Publishers.

Lawler, Jocalyn. 2006. *Behind the Screens: Nursing, Somology, and the Problem of the Body.* Sydney: Sydney University Press.

Leder, Drew. 1990. "Flesh and Blood: A Proposed Supplement to Merleau-Ponty." *Human Studies* 13(3): 209–19.

Locsin, Rozzano C. 2001. *Advancing Technology, Caring and Nursing.* Westport, CT: Auburn House Press.

Lumby, Judy. 1991. *Nursing: Reflecting on an Evolving Practice.* Geelong, Vic.: Deakin University Press.

Lupton, Deborah. 2008. *Medicine as Culture: Illness Disease and the Body*. London: Sage Publishing.

Merleau-Ponty, Maurice. [1945] 1962. *Phenomenology of Perception.* London: Routledge Classics.

Mitchell, Natasha. 2015. "Mental As: Little Acts of Kindness." *ABC Life Matters* (podcast), 9 October. Australian Broadcasting Company. http://mpegmedia.abc.net.au/rn/podcast/2015/10/lms_20151002_0905.mp3.

Murray, Jock. 1995. *Reflections: Images of Illness.* Nova Scotia: Robert Pope Foundation.

Nordenfelt, Lennart, and Per-Erick Liss. 2003. *Dimensions of Health and Health Promotion.* Amsterdam: Rodopi.

"Nurses 'Drowning in a Sea of Paperwork'." 2013. *BBC News*, 21 April.
http://www.bbc.com/news/health-22206882.

O'Doherty, Brian. 2000. *The White Cube: The Ideology of the Gallery Space Expanded Edition.* Los Angeles: University of California Press.

Panda, Sadhu Charan. 2006. "Medicine: Art or Science?" *Mens Sana Monographs* 4(1): 127–38. http://www.ncbi.nlm.nih.gov/pmc/articles/PMC3190445/.

Pearce, Susan M.1994. *Interpreting Objects and Collections.* London: Routledge.

Peloquin, Suzanne M. 1989. "Helping through Touch: The Embodiment of Caring." *Journal of Religion and Health* 8(4) Winter: 299–322.

Pope, Robert. 2004. *Illness and Healing: Images of Cancer.* Nova Scotia: Robert Pope Foundation.

"Rebecca Horn, Finger Gloves, 1972." 2004. *Tate* (website). http://www.tate.org.uk/art/artworks/horn-finger-gloves-t07485.

Rolfe, Gary. 1997. "Beyond Expertise: Theory, Practice and the Reflexive Practitioner." *Journal of Clinical Nursing* 6: 93–97.

Rousselot, Jean, ed. 1967. *Medicine in Art: A Cultural History.* New York: McGraw-Hill Book Company.

Society for the Study of Process Philosophies (website). n.d. Last accessed 15 March 2008. web02.gonzaga.edu/faculty/henning/sspp/.

Sokai, Alan. 2008. *Beyond the Hoax: Science, Philosophy and Culture.* Oxford: Oxford University Press.

Stafford, Barbara Maria. 1997. *Body Criticism: Imaging the Unseen in Enlightenment Art and Medicine.* Cambridge, MA: MIT Press.

Sudjic, Deyan.2008. *The Language of Things.* London: Allen Lane (an imprint of Penguin).

Summers, Sandy. 2008. "Nurse Paintings: Richard Prince." *The Truth about Nursing* (website). http://www.truthaboutnursing.org/media/va/nurse_paintings.html.

Swanbrow, Diane. 1995. "100 Years of a Piercing Glance." *Michigan Today* 27(1). http://deepblue.lib.umich.edu/handle/2027.42/61040.

Turner, Byan S. 2006. "The Body." *Theory Culture and Society* 23(2–3): 223–36.

van der Peet, Rob. 1995. *The Nightingale Model of Nursing.* Edinburgh: Campion Press.

Watkins, Jonathan, ed. 1998. "Introduction." In *Everyday, 11th Biennale of Sydney.* Exhibition catalogue. Sydney: Bloxham and Chambers Pty Ltd.

Watson, Jean. 1985. *Nursing: The Philosophy and Science of Caring.* Boulder: Colorado Associated University Press.

———. 2002. *Assessing and Measuring Caring in Nursing and Health Science.* New York: Springer Publishing Company.

Weil, Simone. 1939. *First and Last Notebooks.* London: Oxford University Press.

Wolf, Zane Robinson. 2013. *Exploring Nursing Rituals: Joining Art and Science.* New York: Springer Publishing Company Inc.

Žižek, Slavoj. 1997. *The Plague of Fantasies.* London: Verso Books.

BIBLIOGRAPHY

Ackerman, Dianne. 1995. *The Natural History of the Senses.* New York: Random House.

Australian Bureau of Statistics. 2013. *Doctors and Nurses Australian Social Trends.*
http://www.abs.gov.au/AUSSTATS/abs@.nfs/Lookup/4102.OMain+Features.

Balls, Paula. 2009. "Phenomenology in Nursing Research: Methodology, Interviewing and Transcribing." *Nursing Times* 105(32–33): 30–33.

Benjamin, Walter. 1936. "The Work of Art in the Age of Mechanical Reproduction." Translated by Harry Zohn. *Marxist Internet Archive.*
marxists.org /reference/subject/philosophy/works/ge/benjamin.htm.

Benner, Patricia, Christine Tanner, and Catherine Chesla. 2009. *Expertise in Nursing Practice.* New York: Springer Publishing Company.

Best, Susan. 2001. "What Is Affect? Considering the Affective Dimension of Contemporary Installation Art." *Australian and New Zealand Journal of Art* 2/3: 207–25.

Bois, Yve-Alain, ed. 2009. *Gabriel Orozco.* Cambridge, MA: MIT Press.

Brush Kidwell, Claudia, and Valerie Steele. 1989. *Men and Women Dressing the Part.* Washington: Smithsonian Institution Press.

Buck-Morss, Susan. 1992. "Aesthetics and Anesthetics: Walter Benjamin's Artwork Essay Reconsidered." *October* 62: 3–41.

Cluff, Leighton E., and Robert Binstock. 2001. *The Lost Art of Caring.* Baltimore: John Hopkins University Press.
Craik, Jennifer. 2005. *Uniform Exposed: From Conformity to Transgression.* Oxford: Berg.

Diprose, Roslyn, and Robyn Ferrell. 1991. *Cartographies: Post structuralism and the Mapping of Bodies and Spaces.* Sydney: Allen & Unwin.

Donahue, Patricia. 1985. *Nursing, The Finest Art: An Illustrated History.* St. Louis, MO: Mosby Company.

Dubroff, M. Dee. 2010. "Japanese Robots Become Hospital Staff." *Weird Asia News*, 13 November.
http://www.weirdasianews.com/2010/11/13japanese-robots-hospital-staff/.

Dyer, Jennifer. 2009. "Review of *The Everyday*, ed. Stephen Johnstone." *Invisible Culture: An Electronic Journal for Visual Culture* 13.
https://www.rochester.edu/in_visible_culture/Issue_13_/reviews/dyer.html.

Ehrenreich, Barbara, and Deirdre English. 1975. *Witches, Midwives, and Nurses, A History of Women Healers.* New York: The Feminist Press.

The Emotive Image of Nursing, The Media Portrayal of the Nurse. 1997. Australia: Waterbyrd Filmz. Video recording.

"Everyday." *Wikipedia*, last updated 13 July 2015. http://enwikipedia.org/wiki/Everyday_life.

Ferrell, Betty, Rose Virani, Hollye Harrington Jacobs, Pam Molloy, and Kathe Kelly. 2010. "Arts and Humanities in Palliative Nursing." *Journal of Pain and Symptom Management* 39(5): 941–45.

Formis, Barbara. 2004. "Event and Readymade: Delayed Sabotage." *Communication and Cognition* 37: 247–61.

Foster, Hal. 1996. *The Return of the Real: The Avant-Garde at the End of the Century.* Cambridge, MA: MIT Press.

Foucault, Michel. 1973. *Birth of the Clinic.* London: Routledge.

Fussell, Paul. 2003. *Uniforms: Why We Are What We Wear.* Boston: Houghton Mifflin Harcourt.

Gendlin, Eugene. 1959. The Focusing Institute Inc. http://www.focusing.org/gendlin/docs/gol_2077.html.

Gregory, Helen, and Cecilia Brazil. 1993. *Bearers of Tradition.* Brisbane: Boolarong Publications.

Grosz, Elizabeth. 1995. *Space, Time and Perversion.* St Leonards, NSW: Allen & Unwin.

Hall, Edward T. 1973. *The Silent Language.* New York: Anchor.

Haynes, Deborah J. 1997. *The Vocation of the Artist.* New York: Cambridge University Press.

Hein, Eleanor. 2001. *Nursing Issues in the 21st Century.* Philadelphia: Lippincott, Williams, and Wilkins.

Hudek, Anthony, ed. 2014. *The Object.* Cambridge, MA: MIT Press.

Hudson-Jones, Anne. 1988. *Images of Nurses: Perspectives from History, Art, and Literature.* Philadelphia: University of Pennsylvania Press.

Johnstone, Stephen, ed. 2008. *The Everyday.* London: Whitechapel Gallery.

Jung, Carl. 1961. *Memories, Dreams and Reflections.* London: Fontana.

Khadra, Mohamed. 2009. *Making the Cut: A Surgeon's Story.* Sydney: Random House.

———. 2010. *Terminal Decline.* Sydney: Random House.

Koh, Germaine. 2005. *Knitwork.*
    http://www.germainekoh.com/ma/projects_details.cfm?pg=projects&projectID==87.

Kossolapow, Line, Sarah Scoble, and Diane Waller, eds. 2003. *Arts – Therapies – Communication.* Berlin: LIT Verlag.

Krysl, Marilyn. 2012. "Writing the Caring Experience." *Marilyn Krysl* (website).
    http://www.marilynkrysl.com/krysl/nursing.html.

Kuhse, Helga. 1997. *Caring: Nurses, Women and Ethics.* Oxford: Blackwell Publishers.

Lawler, Jocalyn. 1997. *The Body in Nursing.* Melbourne, Vic.: Churchill Livingstone.

———. 2006. *Behind the Screens: Nursing, Somology, and the Problem of the Body.* Sydney: Sydney University Press.

Leder, Drew. 1990. "Flesh and Blood: A Proposed Supplement to Merleau-Ponty." *Human Studies* 13(3): 209–19.

Locsin, Rozzano C. 2001. *Advancing Technology, Caring and Nursing.* Westport, CT: Auburn House Press.

Lumby, Judy. 1991. *Nursing: Reflecting on an Evolving Practice.* Geelong, Vic.: Deakin University Press.

Lupton, Deborah. 2008. *Medicine as Culture: Illness Disease and the Body*. London: Sage Publishing.

Manners Norman, G. 1999. *Bullwinkle.* Malven, Vic: Louis Braille. Audio recording.

Massey, Lyle. 2005. "Pregnancy and Pathology: Picturing Childbirth in Eighteenth-Century Obstetric Atlases." *The Art Bulletin* 87(1): 73–91.

McDonnell, Peter and Jean McNiff. 2015. *Action Research for Nurses.* New York: Sage.

Melville, Stephen. 2005. *The Lure of the Object.* Massachusetts: Studley Press.

Merleau-Ponty, Maurice. [1945] 1962. *Phenomenology of Perception.* London: Routledge Classics.

Michalis, Rovithis, R. N. 2002. "Nursing as an Art." *ICUs and Nursing Web Journal.*
    http://www.nursing.gn/Artnursing.pdf.

Mitchell, Natasha. 2015. "Mental As: Little Acts of Kindness." *ABC Life Matters* (podcast), 9
    October. Australian Broadcasting Company.
    http://mpegmedia.abc.net.au/rn/podcast/2015/10/lms_20151002_0905.mp3.

Murray, Jock. 1995. *Reflections: Images of Illness.* Nova Scotia: Robert Pope Foundation.

Neuwirth, Zeen E. 2002. "Reclaiming the Lost Meanings of Medicine." *The Medical Journal of
    Australia* 176(2): 77–79. http://www.mja.com.au/publicissues.

Nordenfelt, Lennart, and Per-Erick Liss. 2003. *Dimensions of Health and Health Promotion.*
    Amsterdam: Rodopi.

"Nurses 'Drowning in a Sea of Paperwork'." 2013. *BBC News*, 21 April.
    http://www.bbc.com/news/health-22206882.

O'Doherty, Brian. 2000. *The White Cube: The Ideology of the Gallery Space Expanded Edition.*
    Los Angeles: University of California Press.

Panda, Sadhu Charan. 2006. "Medicine: Art or Science?" *Mens Sana Monographs* 4(1): 127–38.
    http://www.ncbi.nlm.nih.gov/pmc/articles/PMC3190445/.

Pearce, Susan M.1994. *Interpreting Objects and Collections.* London: Routledge.

Peloquin, Suzanne M. 1989. "Helping through Touch: The Embodiment of Caring." *Journal of
    Religion and Health* 8(4) Winter: 299–322.

Pope, Robert. 2004. *Illness and Healing: Images of Cancer.* Nova Scotia: Robert Pope
    Foundation.

Pratt, Michael, and Anat Rafaeli. 1997. "Organizational Dress as a Symbol of Multilayered
    Social Identities." *Academy of Management Journal* 40(4): 862–98.

"Rebecca Horn, Finger Gloves, 1972." 2004. *Tate* (website).
    http://www.tate.org.uk/art/artworks/horn-finger-gloves-t07485.

Roberts, Joan, and Thetis M. Group. 1995. *Feminism and Nursing.* Westport, CT: Praeger
    Publishing,

Rogers, Nanette. 2005. *The Proper Nurse.* Burleigh, Qld: Zeus Publications.

Rolfe, Gary. 1997. "Beyond Expertise: Theory, Practice and the Reflexive Practitioner." *Journal
    of Clinical Nursing* 6: 93–97.

Rousselot, Jean, ed. 1967. *Medicine in Art: A Cultural History.* New York: McGraw-Hill Book
    Company.

Society for the Study of Process Philosophies (website). n.d. Last accessed 15 March 2008. web02.gonzaga.edu/faculty/henning/sspp/.

Soderqvist, Thomas. 2007. "Exploring and Curating Medical Objects with the Sense of Touch." *Medical Museoin* (website), 20 September. http://www.museion.ku.dk/2007/09/exploring-and-curating-medical-objects-with-the-sense-of-touch/.

Sokai, Alan. 2008. *Beyond the Hoax: Science, Philosophy and Culture.* Oxford: Oxford University Press.

Spragley, F., & F. Francis. 2006. "Nursing Uniforms: Professional Symbol or Outdated Relic?" *Nursing Management* 37(10): 55–58.

Stafford, Barbara Maria. 1997. *Body Criticism: Imaging the Unseen in Enlightenment Art and Medicine.* Cambridge, MA: MIT Press.

Stafford, Barbara Maria, and Frances Terpak. 2001. *Devices of Wonder: From the World in a Box to Images on a Screen.* Los Angeles: Getty Research Institute. Cambridge, MA: MIT Press.

Staricoff, Rosalia Lechukst. 2004. Arts Council of England, Report 36. *Arts in Health: A Review of the Medical Literature.* http://www.yaq.org.au/wp-content/uploads2013/06staricoff.

Stewart, David, and Algis Mickunas. 1990. *Exploring Phenomenology.* Athens, Greece: Ohio University Press.

Sudjic, Deyan.2008. *The Language of Things.* London: Allen Lane (an imprint of Penguin).

Summers, Sandy. 2008. "Nurse Paintings: Richard Prince." *The Truth about Nursing* (website). http://www.truthaboutnursing.org/media/va/nurse_paintings.html.

Swanbrow, Diane. 1995. "100 Years of a Piercing Glance." *Michigan Today* 27(1). http://deepblue.lib.umich.edu/handle/2027.42/61040.

Taylor, Beverly J. 1994. *Ordinariness in Nursing.* Melbourne: Churchill Livingstone.

Trilling, James. 2001. *The Language of Ornament.* London: Thames and Hudson.

Turner, Byan S. 2006. "The Body." *Theory Culture and Society* 23(2–3): 223–36.

van der Peet, Rob. 1995. *The Nightingale Model of Nursing.* Edinburgh: Campion Press.

Watkins, Jonathan, ed. 1998. "Introduction." In *Everyday, 11th Biennale of Sydney.* Exhibition catalogue. Sydney: Bloxham and Chambers Pty Ltd.

Watson, Jean. 1985. *Nursing: The Philosophy and Science of Caring.* Boulder: Colorado Associated University Press.

———. 2002. *Assessing and Measuring Caring in Nursing and Health Science.* New York: Springer Publishing Company.

Weil, Simone. 1939. *First and Last Notebooks.* London: Oxford University Press.

Wickstrom Brit-Maj. 2004. "Nursing Education at an Art Gallery." *Journal of Nursing Scholarship* 32(2): 197–99.

Wolf, Zane Robinson. 1988. *Nurses' Work: The Sacred and the Profane.* Philadelphia: University of Pennsylvania Press.

———. 2013. *Exploring Nursing Rituals: Joining Art and Science.* New York: Springer Publishing Company Inc.

Žižek, Slavoj. 1997. *The Plague of Fantasies.* London: Verso Books.

Zwerdling, Michael. 2004. *Postcards of Nursing: A Worldwide Tribute.* Philadelphia: Lippincott Williams and Wilkins.

Cover Image:
Deep Listening
a watercolour by Hazel Mary Cope

Cover design by John Thiessen